EXPERIENCING ACT FROM THE INSIDE OUT

SELF-PRACTICE/SELF-REFLECTION GUIDES FOR PSYCHOTHERAPISTS

James Bennett-Levy, Series Editor

This series invites therapists to enhance their effectiveness "from the inside out" using self-practice/self-reflection (SP/SR). Books in the series lead therapists through a structured three-stage process of focusing on a personal or professional issue they want to change, practicing therapeutic techniques on themselves (self-practice), and reflecting on the experience (self-reflection). Research supports the unique benefits of SP/SR for providing insights and skills not readily available through more conventional training procedures. The approach is suitable for therapists at all levels of experience, from trainees to experienced supervisors. Series volumes have a large-size format for ease of use and feature reproducible worksheets and forms that purchasers can download and print.

Experiencing CBT from the Inside Out:
A Self-Practice/Self-Reflection Workbook for Therapists
James Bennett-Levy, Richard Thwaites, Beverly Haarhoff, and Helen Perry

Experiencing Schema Therapy from the Inside Out:
A Self-Practice/Self-Reflection Workbook for Therapists
Joan M. Farrell and Ida A. Shaw

Experiencing Compassion-Focused Therapy from the Inside Out:
A Self-Practice/Self-Reflection Workbook for Therapists
Russell L. Kolts, Tobyn Bell, James Bennett-Levy, and Chris Irons

Experiencing ACT from the Inside Out:
A Self-Practice/Self-Reflection Workbook for Therapists
Dennis Tirch, Laura R. Silberstein-Tirch, R. Trent Codd, III,
Martin J. Brock, and M. Joann Wright

Experiencing ACT from the Inside Out

A Self-Practice/Self-Reflection Workbook for Therapists

Dennis Tirch
Laura R. Silberstein-Tirch
R. Trent Codd, III
Martin J. Brock
M. Joann Wright

Series Editor's Note by James Bennett-Levy

THE GUILFORD PRESS
New York   London

Copyright © 2019 The Guilford Press
A Division of Guilford Publications, Inc.
370 Seventh Avenue, Suite 1200, New York, NY 10001
www.guilford.com

Printed in the United States of America

This book is printed on acid-free paper.

Last digit is print number: 9   8   7   6   5   4   3   2   1

The authors have checked with sources believed to be reliable in their efforts to provide information
that is complete and generally in accord with the standards of practice that are accepted at the time of
publication. However, in view of the possibility of human error or changes in behavioral, mental health,
or medical sciences, neither the authors, nor the editor and publisher, nor any other party who has been
involved in the preparation or publication of this work warrants that the information contained herein
is in every respect accurate or complete, and they are not responsible for any errors or omissions or the
results obtained from the use of such information. Readers are encouraged to confirm the information
contained in this book with other sources.

Library of Congress Cataloging-in-Publication Data

Names: Tirch, Dennis D., 1968– author.
Title: Experiencing ACT from the inside out : a self-practice/self-reflection workbook for therapists /
    Dennis Tirch [and 4 others].
Description: New York : The Guilford Press, [2019] | Series: Self-practice/self-reflection guides for
    psychotherapists | Includes bibliographical references and index.
Identifiers: LCCN 2019004363| ISBN 9781462540648 (paperback) | ISBN 9781462540655 (hardcover)
Subjects: LCSH: Acceptance and commitment therapy—Handbooks, manuals, etc. | BISAC:
    MEDICAL / Psychiatry / General. | SOCIAL SCIENCE / Social Work.
Classification: LCC RC489.A32 T573 2019 | DDC 616.89/1425—dc23
LC record available at *https://lccn.loc.gov/2019004363*

About the Authors

Dennis Tirch, PhD, is founder of the Center for Compassion Focused Therapy in New York City and Associate Clinical Professor in the Icahn School of Medicine at Mt. Sinai Medical Center. He is author or coauthor of numerous books, chapters, and peer-reviewed articles on acceptance and commitment therapy (ACT), compassion-focused therapy (CFT), cognitive-behavioral therapy (CBT), and Buddhist psychology. His books include *Buddhist Psychology and Cognitive-Behavioral Therapy* and *Emotion Regulation in Psychotherapy*. Dr. Tirch is president of the Association for Contextual Behavioral Science (ACBS) and the Compassionate Mind Foundation USA. He provides online and in-person workshops and trainings globally in mindfulness-, compassion-, and acceptance-based interventions. Dr. Tirch is a Fellow of ACBS and a Fellow and Certified Trainer/Consultant of the Academy of Cognitive Therapy. He is a Dharma Holder and teacher in the Zen Garland lineage.

Laura R. Silberstein-Tirch, PsyD, is Director of the Center for Compassion Focused Therapy and Adjunct Assistant Professor at Albert Einstein College of Medicine of Yeshiva University. She is a clinical supervisor and CFT trainer who presents internationally on mindfulness and compassion. She is coauthor of books including *Buddhist Psychology and Cognitive-Behavioral Therapy*. Dr. Silberstein-Tirch is president of the New York City chapter of ACBS and Executive Director of the Compassionate Mind Foundation USA. Her research interests include psychological flexibility and emotions as well as CFT for anxiety and depression.

R. Trent Codd, III, EdS, BCBA, is Executive Director of the Cognitive-Behavioral Therapy Center of Western North Carolina in Asheville, where he treats a broad range of clinical concerns. He has particular interest in refractory depression and obsessive–compulsive spectrum disorders. Mr. Codd is a charter member of ACBS and a Fellow and Trainer/Consultant of the Academy of Cognitive Therapy. He is coauthor of

Teaching and Supervising Cognitive Behavioral Therapy and editor of *Practice-Based Research: A Guide for Clinicians.*

Martin J. Brock, MSc, MA, RMN, is Senior Lecturer in the Department of Counselling and Psychotherapy and Program Leader for the Postgraduate Certificate in Compassion Focused Therapy at the University of Derby, United Kingdom. He has had a long career in the National Health Service in the United Kingdom, practicing and supervising evidence-based psychotherapies. Mr. Brock has advanced training and experience in CBT, mindfulness-based CBT, CFT, and ACT. He has served as president of the United Kingdom and Republic of Ireland chapter of ACBS; was a founding member of the British Association for Behavioural and Cognitive Psychotherapies ACT special interest group; and was the first peer-reviewed ACT trainer in the United Kingdom. As an ACT trainer and supervisor, Mr. Brock has regularly delivered workshops globally since 2006.

M. Joann Wright, PhD, is a clinical psychologist with the Linden Oaks Medical Group in Naperville, Illinois. She is a peer-reviewed trainer in ACT and a Fellow of ACBS. Dr. Wright has provided ACT training to doctoral students and therapists nationally and internationally since 2008. She is dedicated to teaching and delivering ACT to help people reduce suffering in their lives. She is coauthor of *Learning ACT for Group Treatment: An Acceptance and Commitment Therapy Skills Training Manual for Therapists.*

Series Editor's Note

Experiencing ACT from the Inside Out is the fourth book in The Guilford Press Self-Practice/Self-Reflection Guides for Psychotherapists series. Many therapists have told me how much they have been looking forward to the publication of this book. They will not be disappointed.

These five authors have done a wonderful job in creating a self-practice/self-reflection (SP/SR) workbook that will appeal to both novice and experienced therapists. For new therapists, it puts flesh and muscle on the bones of conceptual understanding. For experienced therapists, it offers the richest of paths to deepen awareness and understanding of both their "personal self" and their "therapist self." As either a novice or an experienced accceptance and commitment therapy (ACT) therapist, you will notice a significant increase in your therapeutic skills through experiencing and reflecting on the exercises in this book.

Choosing the authors for the ACT SP/SR book was not a difficult task. One person stood out: Dennis Tirch. By the time I experienced Dennis's teaching for the first time in 2013, he had already cowritten three books, with two more on the drawing board. At that workshop in Byron Bay, Australia, in 2013, cofacilitated with Paul Gilbert, I immediately recognized a workshop leader who led participants seamlessly into experiential activities. Dennis walked the talk. I already knew that he was a compelling writer as well, so the choice was simple. In turn, Dennis assembled a team of colleagues who shared his vision and were committed to try out all the activities in the book for themselves. As you will experience, the results are awe-inspiring. The honesty and courage of Dennis, Laura, Trent, Martin, and Joann shines through their self-practice examples and self-reflections during a period of writing in which they were confronted with some truly difficult experiences.

A few words about SP/SR in the context of ACT. It is central to the practice of ACT that we learn through experiencing and that avoidance of our internal experience will often result in greater suffering. This understanding applies as much to therapists' experience as to clients. However, therapists' avoidance of internal experience creates an additional problem in the context of client work. It may result in their missing important cues about their own well-being, as well as the well-being of their clients. So there is a particular need for therapists to be as open, accepting, and flexible with their experience as they can.

The SP/SR examples provided by these five authors are a testament to the ACT values of acceptance, compassion, and committed action, sometimes in the face of considerable adversity. One word of warning though: Do not feel that you have to choose the same issues for your SP/SR as those that confronted these authors! In previous SP/SR workbooks, we suggested that participants in SP/SR programs choose issues of mild to moderate emotional intensity, but not major—typically something with an intensity rating of 40–75%. The point is to avoid feeling so overwhelmed in your learning journey that you cannot focus on deepening your ACT skills. If your primary purpose in doing SP/SR is therapist skill development, we would suggest choosing a professional or personal issue to work with in this midrange.

A second point about SP/SR. What we have learned through the SP/SR journey is that experiencing is only half the story. Reflecting on experience is the other half. Through reflection, we bring to mind our experience. Then we engage in what is probably a unique human capacity: the capacity for new learning without any additional external input. By bringing our experience to mind again, embodying it, and asking carefully constructed reflective questions about our experience, we can not only revisit the original experience, but derive new insights and understandings that were unavailable at the time. This is the power of reflection.

In this book, you will find carefully crafted self-reflective questions at the end of each module. The authors suggest that you write your reflections. This is purposeful. We have found over the 20 years of SP/SR work that there is a huge difference between "reflecting in your head" and written reflections. You will notice two things. First, written reflections take time, energy, and effort. Second, the time, energy, and effort are rewarded many times over by additional insights and development of a skill set that will deepen your experience of yourself and your relationships, personally and professionally.

It is with great pleasure that I commend this admirable book to the reader, though "reader" is the wrong word in the SP/SR context. If you just read the book, you will miss the point of it, and miss out on the vast majority of the learning. So let me rephrase: It is with great pleasure that I commend this admirable book to the ACT experiencer and self-reflector.

JAMES BENNETT-LEVY

Acknowledgments

Dennis Tirch and Laura R. Silberstein-Tirch: We are both honored and moved to have been able to work with our beloved friends Trent, Martin, and Joann on a project that truly shaped our lives together. James Bennett-Levy is our spiritual brother, and his brilliant self-practice/self-reflection (SP/SR) work is just an outward emanation of the brilliance of his heart-mind. Our editor, Kitty Moore, is a hero to us, in her compassion, cleverness, and wit, and we are deeply grateful to her. The entire team at Guilford were hugely supportive. We would like to acknowledge and honor our many friends, colleagues, teachers, and mentors—all of whom have influenced who we are and the work we do—especially Steven C. Hayes, Kelly Wilson, Robert L. Leahy, Paul Gilbert, Erica Silberstein, Robert Fripp, Lata McGinn, Sara Reichenbach Manor, Philp Inwood, Aisling Curtin, Louise McHugh, Roshi Paul Genki Kahn, Roshi Monika Genmitsu Kahn, Sensei Cathleen Kanno Dowd, Kristin Neff, Chris Germer, Racheli Miller, Geoffrey Gold, Noel Taylor, Frank Bond, Emanuele Rossi, Chris Irons, Korina Ioannou, Lisa Coyne, Evelyn Gould, Nanni Presti, Russell Kolts, Robyn Walser, Louise Hayes, Jonathan Bricker, Amy Murrell, D. J. Moran, Nic Hooper, Mark Sisti, James Kirby, Stan Steindl, Haley Quinn, Joseph LeDoux, Stefan Hofman, Arthur Freeman, Nicola Petrocchi, Marcela Matos, Yotam Heineberg, Russ Harris, Sonja Batten, Miranda Morris, Amy House, Emily Sandoz, Kate Kellum, Priscilla Almada, Jessica Dore, Jim Campilongo, Ross White, David Gillanders, Timothy Gordon, Troy DuFrene, Heather Garnos, Rikke Kjelgaard, Mie Tastesen, Francis Gheysen, Kimberly Sogge, Tom Szabo, Nancy Ring, Chris Fraser, Linda Hamilton, ChiaYing Chou, Mary Sawyer, Maria Karekla, Andreas B. Larsson, Barry Sanders, Tina Siragusa, Sandra Georgescu, Owen Rachel, Jennifer Villatte, Matthieu Villatte, Carrie Diamond, Emily Rodrigues, Stephen K. Hayes, Richard Sears, Lauren Whitelaw, Theresa Robertson, and Tom Borkovec. We also thank our extended family: Auferio, Barnwell, Ewig, Flax, Fritz, Kondo, Lonegan, Parany, Samuels, Simpson, and Young; Dennis's stepfather, Neal Tanis, who flew away while this book was being written; our much beloved Silberstein and Tirch families;

and, most importantly, our daughter, Cassidy Dharma Rain Tirch, who arrived while this book was in development!

R. Trent Codd, III: Dennis and Laura visited me in my hometown of Asheville, North Carolina, in September 2014. During that visit they asked me whether I'd be interested in coauthoring a book on ACT SP/SR with them. Saying yes to working with two close friends on a meaningful venture was easy. Little did I know how consequential this project would be for me personally. Dennis and Laura, thank you for inviting me to participate in this journey with you. Martin and Joann, two emotionally brave and beautiful human beings, thank you for your deep friendships. Though there are too many to name, I would like to express gratitude to all who contributed to my development as an ACT therapist. I especially acknowledge and thank Steve Hayes, Kirk Strosahl, and Kelly Wilson. They were always accessible when I had questions and shared their knowledge freely. I would also like to acknowledge, in no particular order, Scott Temple, Cliff Notarius, Rob Zettle, Hank Robb, Jason Luoma, Mike Twohig, Doug Woods, Pat Friman, Jodi Polaha, Martin Ivancic, Allen Cooley (who, sadly, is no longer with us), Amy Murrell, Chad Drake, Christeine Terry, Mike Femenella, Rainer Sonntag, Tom Szabo, and D. J. Moran. Thank you for playing a part in building my ACT repertoire and, more importantly, for being good friends.

Martin J. Brock: I should like to express my deep gratitude to my wonderful coauthors, Dennis, Laura, Trent, and Joann. This has been quite a journey together and I am much the richer for the kindness, wisdom, and inspiration I have received from such brilliant and gifted human beings. Dennis, you inspire all those around you and you have touched so many people in so many ways. I have learned so much from you and am humbled to count you as a brother. Laura, you are so fierce and passionate in all that you do, and you have done so much to advance our understanding of women's lives. Trent, so modest and unassuming but so knowledgeable and so generous of your time and energy. I look forward to spending more time in your gentle light. Joann, you enriched our journey so much with your enthusiasm and passion, but more so with the courage to keep going with our work despite facing tremendous challenges. I acknowledge the many teachers who have guided me along the way and blessed me with their insights, including Robert Leahy, Mark Williams, Melanie Fennell, Steven Hayes, Kirk Strosahl, Sonja Batten, Robyn Walser, and Paul Gilbert—their vision and dedication lit many paths for me. Most of all, I acknowledge the teachings of Kelly Wilson, and more so his willingness to reach out to me in my darkest of times, a truly compassionate and gifted teacher. I should also like to acknowledge the support of dear friends whom I have been honored to know, particularly Mary Sawyer and Sandra Georgescu—you have given me so much more than you may realize. Finally, I acknowledge the gift of family that has made me the man that I am. Linda, An-Marie, and Susan, who shared my first steps on this planet, the connections we have will never fade. Margo, you are my rock and my soulmate, and you gifted me with two of the rarest jewels, our dear daughters, Hanneke and Becky. I am forever in your debt and we will walk together always. Hanneke, you have become one of my biggest teachers and I am in awe of all that you have achieved. For one so young you possess a wisdom and courage that is truly inspirational. Becky, you continue to inspire me to be a better man and to do the best I can in the service of others, and my contribution to this book is testament to that.

M. Joann Wright: I am deeply grateful to my coauthors for inviting me on this remarkable journey of self-discovery that took place in the context of a profound brother- and sisterhood. In addition to your indelible friendships, you all created a very safe space to share vulnerability and love and it was a voyage that will forever shape my life for the better. Namaste. The foundations of my understanding of ACT started with my grad school mentor Joseph R. Scardapane. Joe, this ride began with you. Thank you. My brother-from-another-mother D. J. Moran has served as a mentor and dear friend for decades. I would not be much of an ACT practitioner or the person I am without his influence in my life. I have received such profound and scholarly training from a number of practitioners who served to deepen my understanding of ACT from wise perspectives that at times eluded me: Darrah Westrup, Steve Hayes, Kelly Wilson, Robyn Walser, Sonja Batten, Frank Bond, Kirk Strosahl, Louise Hayes, and Louise McHugh, I thank you for your wisdom and guidance. I thank the Association for Contextual and Behavioral Science for creating such a vibrant scientific and clinical community that brings together the world's finest ACT-informed people to share our research findings and new forms of treatment. You are my intellectual home and family, for which I am powerfully grateful. My supervisees, students, and clients who teach me every day how to do ACT better—you will truly never know how you shaped the way I work. Bless you. Finally, I bow with gratitude to my family and friends—who put the wind in my sails and set me forth in the world with boundless sustenance. My brother, J, and sister, Jan, and our dearly departed parents, who gave me the confidence to dream big—I am very thankful for you. My stepsons, Andrew and Marcus, add joy and remind me to be curious every day. Thank you. You both amaze me. My husband, Larry, who serves as the rock in my life and allows me to roam life's terrain unfettered knowing I will always land in the safety of his love—life would not be as rich without you. I love you.

Contents

PART I

The ACT SP/SR Approach

CHAPTER 1

Introducing *Experiencing ACT from the Inside Out*

Acceptance and commitment therapy (ACT; Hayes, Strosahl, & Wilson, 1999, 2012) is designed from the ground up to bring our best understanding of behavioral science to the problem of human suffering. Through a range of evidence-based techniques ACT emphasizes mindful behavior change and movement toward valued aims as core principles (Hayes, Luoma, Bond, Masuda, & Lillis, 2006). Over the last 20 years, a substantial body of research has demonstrated the effectiveness of ACT interventions across a range of human psychological and medical problems (Hooper & Larsson, 2015).

During that same time, research has demonstrated that psychotherapists' self-practice and self-reflection (SP/SR) training can have a positive impact on therapist development across every experience level (Bennett-Levy & Lee, 2014; Bennett-Levy, Thwaites, Haarhoff, & Perry, 2015). Accordingly, this book is designed *to apply SP/ SR methods to the training of ACT therapists*. Essentially, you can use this workbook as an experiential immersion in the foundational elements of ACT. This means that experienced ACT therapists can work through these exercises and concepts, alone or in a group, to sharpen and deepen their ACT practice. Furthermore, the workbook can serve as an "inside-out" introductory text for beginning ACT therapists.

Not too long ago, the five of us set off on our own ACT SP/SR journey, encountering the methods and processes with which you will be working. It was a transformational experience for each of us. Even though we were all experienced ACT therapists, facing our own problems through ACT SP/SR involved vulnerability and radical honesty. During the time that it took to work through ACT SP/SR and to write this book, we faced some of the most challenging events in our lives. Together we encountered a range of life experiences—traumatic losses and new beginnings, serious illnesses and dramatic recoveries, professional stressors and personal leaps forward—the spectrum of human challenges that Jon Kabat-Zinn (2013) refers to in *Full Catastrophe Living*. During this time, our ACT SP/SR work and our relationships with one another provided us with strength, enhanced perspective, and support.

As a result of our own meaningful experiences practicing ACT from the inside out, we decided that we would use our own problem formulations and observations, rather than use composite characters or fictionalized examples in this book. We are aiming to "walk the walk" here, by introducing you to the reality of our own struggles and our own aspirations. We hope that this creates a context of openness, compassion, and connection as you set off to face similar challenges and opportunities to those we approached.

By engaging in these self-training practices, we hope you will cultivate greater reflective capacity, psychotherapy skills, and a deeper understanding of ACT. Rather than this solely being a book about acquiring knowledge, we have worked to provide a systematic series of exercises and reflections that can facilitate growth in both personal and professional areas of life. Our hope is that this will contribute to your well-being and to the growth and wellness of your clients.

We begin by providing an introduction to the essential rationale of ACT and SP/SR. We then provide some basic guidelines for how to approach this book. Chapters 2–4 provide further foundational material for you on your journey through experiencing ACT from the inside out.

The Aim of ACT SP/SR: Being Open, Centered, and Engaged

ACT is grounded in an appreciation of how we humans are set up for suffering and dissatisfaction by the very nature of human existence and by the dynamic processes embedded in human language and cognition. For example, even under the best of circumstances, much of our day-to-day behavior can seem guided by an "autopilot" mode of action. As we go about our daily tasks, perhaps checking things off our "to-do" list, repeating our habitual patterns of behavior, things might not feel very driven by purpose. If we wish to lose weight, we still might cave in to our urges and eat that second (third?) piece of pizza. Though we desperately long for deeper connections with our friends and family, we still avoid sending that email or planning a weekend together. Sometimes, our behavioral rigidity involves much darker and more painful dimensions. We can't stop ourselves from descending into opiate addiction or finding other escape routes to push away our feelings. We may stay in bed for days due to the weight of our depression, living smaller lives. The momentum of our behavior seems to carry us, unaware, to the next day's actions, like a wave inexorably heading toward the shore. ACT provides us with mindfulness-based interventions that can help us to "wake up" from this autopilot mode of operating. Mindfulness can provide us the space to choose new directions, possibly breaking chains of behavioral rigidity. ACT SP/SR can help us to learn how to feel "centered" in mindful awareness, grounded in this very moment, and ready to take action.

Beyond the routine and inflexible patterns of our actions, our thoughts themselves can also give us a lot of trouble. A great deal of our time can be spent in struggles with emotional pain and negative thoughts. We listen to our inner critic recite the litany of our failures as we distractedly go about our business. We worry about all of the things that could go wrong, imagining potential financial disasters, relationship breakups, or problems within our families. When these imaginary disasters and scolding inner voices show up, we feel them as though they were all too real. Images of failure and tragedy can set our hearts racing. Ironically, the more we try to suppress this kind of thinking, the worse it tends to get, and our efforts to avoid these thoughts only lead us to more intense spirals of feeling threatened and inadequate (Hooper, Saunders, & McHugh, 2010). But it doesn't have to be this way. We don't have to live robotically, and our minds don't need to feel like minefields. ACT involves methods for seeing thoughts and mental events clearly, as what they are and *not what they say they are* (Hayes et al., 1999). By training ourselves to know the difference between real-world situations and the demands of our minds, we may become better able to face the actual challenges and opportunities of life (Deacon, 2011). ACT SP/SR involves training in how to remain "open" to mental events, and how to thereby free ourselves from their excessive influence.

From a foundation of mindful awareness, noticing and accepting the flow of mental events that constantly pulls at our attention, ACT invites us to become the author of valued directions in our lives (Dahl, Plumb, Stewart, & Lundgren, 2009). When we have woken up to the moment, shaken off the cobwebs of mental projections, and set a course for valued living, we may be able to dedicate ourselves to living with greater purpose and meaning. What is it like when we feel that our lives are focused on what matters most? How do we feel when we know that our struggles are a part of moving toward a life that is worth working for, worth suffering for?

Beneath our patterns of automatic responding and our battles within ourselves we can envision some qualities of "doing" or "being" that we wish to bring into the world more fully. We wish to know meaning. We wish to stand for something. If we allow ourselves to quiet the mind and slow the body, turning in kindness to what matters most in this lifetime, we can envision living with purpose and vitality. For example, we might want to be more caring parents. At times, we might hope to become a better partner, or a more responsive friend. Some of us might feel driven to create great art. Establishing financial security might serve as a "true north" compass point for many of us. For those on a more contemplative or spiritual path, daily actions might be guided by the pursuit of personal awakening. Some of us might work to approach our relationships as the Bible tells us Jesus Christ would, aiming to extend love even to those who would seek to harm us. Perhaps we earnestly hope to develop more discipline in our approach to exercise. The range of values that we might carry with us and aspire to realize is as diverse as we are. Whatever your freely chosen values may be, ACT SP/SR involves methods to train ourselves to be "engaged" in our lives, with a commitment to becoming the version of ourselves we most wish to be.

The qualities of being open, centered, and engaged are not just clever ideas in ACT SP/SR. These three "pillars" of our ACT SP/SR practice reflect evidence-based processes and procedures that we can use with our clients in experiential psychotherapy (Hayes et al., 2012). They also represent core processes that we can activate in our personal and professional development, which is one of the goals of the program we share with you in this book. Taken together, being open, centered, and engaged is described as "psychological flexibility." Research has established that cultivating psychological flexibility is key to overcoming a range of psychological problems and to establishing greater well-being (Powers, Zum Vorde Sive Vörding, & Emmelkamp, 2009; Ruiz,

2010). Developing greater psychological flexibility through ACT SP/SR is at the heart of our journey together.

What Is ACT SP/SR?

Consistent with the ACT model, this book focuses on how therapists can breathe life into the pursuit of their valued aims with greater flexibility, compassion, and courage through a systematic and evidence-based SP/SR approach. ACT SP/SR is a structured, experiential training method that involves using ACT techniques on ourselves through self-practice (SP) and of reflecting on that experience through written self-reflection (SR). Through ACT SP/SR, we apply our psychotherapy approach to our own challenges in our personal and professional lives. Of course, any ACT training will involve time focusing on ourselves. Indeed, a great deal of foundational ACT workshop-based training involves experiencing ACT processes in ourselves. ACT SP/SR invites us to devote some time and attention to specifically and methodically deepening our ACT practice by using ACT techniques on ourselves.

Through ACT SP/SR we become our own therapist, sometimes in the company of trusted and caring colleagues who are sharing this journey. In order to structure and organize the inner work undertaken with this workbook, *we are asking you to choose a specific problem or domain of action to focus on during your work in this ACT SP/ SR program*. This can be a problem in your professional or personal life, or perhaps an issue that spans both of these aspects of your world. After engaging in each period of ACT SP, you will take time to engage in SR about your work and lived experience. These reflections appear to be more meaningful and impactful if they are written down, rather than just articulated out loud or even spoken "in our heads" (Bennett-Levy & Lee, 2014; Bennett-Levy, Lee, Travers, Pohlman, & Hamernik, 2003). These reflections involve many levels of application, doing, and being. For example, after practicing radical acceptance techniques around a distressing emotion, we might reflect upon the meaning of our experience for ourselves, for our work with clients, or even what implications our insights might have for ACT theory and practice.

ACT SP/SR work can be done as an individual practice. Indeed, readers of this book will likely more often be practicing on their own, working through these techniques as a part of their ongoing education and inner work. Importantly, SP/SR work can also take place in a group. Much of the research on SP/SR work took place in a group context (Bennett-Levy, McManus, Westling, & Fennell, 2009)—we formed just such a group as we developed this approach. In this context, we weren't serving as a support group or therapy group or providing therapy to one another—rather, we were working on ourselves in the context of a supportive and trusted community of friends. The research tells us that SP/SR participants have often reported a "deeper sense of knowing the therapy" (Bennett-Levy et al., 2015; Thwaites et al., 2015). We also shared this observation during a meaningful period of work. Candidly, this work lifted us up during some difficult times, and it helped us know our work and ourselves better while learning ACT from the inside out.

Why ACT SP/SR?

In a sense, the SP/SR method and the development of ACT are both extensions of a seismic change in the zeitgeist of the cognitive-behavioral tradition, sometimes described as a "third wave" (Hayes, 2004). This shift of emphasis away from mechanistic models and toward methods that embraced experiential and reflective practice began near the end of the 20th century and has continued into the first decades of the 21st century (Tirch, Silberstein, & Kolts, 2015). While early cognitive-behavioral therapy (CBT) training did not involve much explicit emphasis on the exploration of the therapist's own process, SP/SR method developer James Bennett-Levy (personal communication, August 13, 2018) has noted that a significant trend toward appreciation of interpersonal process and self-exploration emerged within CBT in the mid-1990s, contributing to the development of the SP/SR approach. SP/SR was designed as a training strategy to enhance the development of therapists' skills through practicing therapy techniques on themselves and engaging in SR from both a personal and professional perspective (Bennett-Levy et al., 2001).

The SP/SR approach became a part of a growing body of research within traditional CBT that emphasized and examined self-experience and SR. During roughly this time period, ACT and the contextual movement within the behavioral sciences also flourished and spread rapidly. With an emphasis on mindfulness, acceptance, and compassion, ACT naturally emphasized self-exploration, though using a different series of techniques. Accordingly, you are likely to find that integrating an SP/SR approach into ACT can be a much smoother transition than you might expect.

The growing body of SP/SR research demonstrates that this form of training allows us to develop greater attunement in the interpersonal dimension of the psychotherapy relationship (Gale & Schröder, 2014; Thwaites et al., 2015). Therapists who have completed SP/SR training have reported growth in important dimensions of the therapy relationship, including empathic understanding, therapeutic presence, and compassion (Gale & Schröder, 2014; Spendelow & Butler, 2016; Thwaites et al., 2015). These SP/SR research findings have been found across countries, groups, and levels of experience (Bennett-Levy, 2019). Additionally, psychotherapists have reported greater self-confidence and confidence in their therapy approach after training in SP/SR (Gale & Schröder, 2014). This has involved therapists reporting an enhancement of both their conceptual skills and technical skills after taking part in SP/SR training.

Pakenham (2015) has repeatedly explored the value of self-care and ACT SP, with a particular emphasis on dealing with the impact of stress during graduate training. While this research does not follow a manualized SP/SR protocol, it has pioneered the use of the ACT model for personal practice. Based on a review of the literature, Pakenham and Stafford-Brown (2012) note that high levels of stress and potential burnout among clinicians have not been adequately addressed by current training models. Their group has put forward a call to arms for the field, suggesting the implementation of mindfulness- and acceptance-based methods consistent with our ACT SP/SR approach (Stafford-Brown & Pakenham, 2012). Using a "self-as-laboratory" approach, Pakenham and his colleagues examined the impact of ACT training and SP in several studies involving clinical psychology trainees. Their research reported that participants had significant improvements in mindfulness, specific therapist skills, increased psychological flexibility, and decreased personal distress. Thus far, research in the ACT work has mirrored the findings of research using SP/SR among CBT practitioners and suggests the value of learning ACT from the inside out, in the way we elaborate in this workbook.

Orientation to *Experiencing ACT from the Inside Out*

This book is divided into two parts. The first main section includes the foundational chapters that explain our approach and help you prepare to engage in the practical work that follows throughout our ACT SP/SR method. We suggest that everyone using this book should read Chapters 1–3. Chapters 1 and 2 provide the theoretical orientation and conceptual foundation for ACT SP/SR. Some of you who are more familiar with the underlying philosophy of science, theory of cognition, and therapy method involved in ACT might find these two earlier chapters to be a review. *Nonetheless, we invite you to return to this material with fresh eyes and a "beginner's mind" as much as you can as you begin your ACT SP/SR journey.* If you can, put yourself in the place of your client or an early career therapist and begin to engage with this material from a fresh perspective.

One of the central concerns in the ACT community involves approaching ACT as a model of applied contextual behavioral science rather than as a toolbox of psychotherapy techniques. ACT was never intended to be adopted merely as a therapy protocol, but was designed and developed as a scalable model for cultivating well-being grounded in evidence-based processes and principles. Understanding the underlying philosophy and conceptual model that supports ACT is *the key* to using ACT techniques effectively. For this reason, we highly suggest working with the material in the introductory chapters and responding to the reflective questions that are included. The best ACT therapists we know use their mastery of basic behavioral principles to improvise and develop new interventions that are sensitive to real-time contingencies that they encounter with their clients. Our hope is that your review and engagement with this material will help you hone these skills through your SP/SR journey.

Chapter 3 provides guidelines and suggestions for any person participating in an ACT SP/SR group. This chapter will help you consider practical considerations, such as whether it will be best to practice on your own or with a group. The chapter offers suggestions about how you might identify and understand the problem you are choosing to work on as you use this ACT SP/SR workbook. Additionally, the chapter provides further information about how to best approach SR and how to bridge among our personal practice, reflection, and application.

Chapter 3 also prepares you to use the practice-based components of the book that are organized as "modules." The modules each reflect the processes that interact to bring forth and enhance psychological flexibility. Furthermore, the modules build on the psychological flexibility model to help us bring greater mindfulness and self-compassion into our work with ourselves as psychotherapeutic instruments. While it might seem easy, and even tempting, to breeze through the modules by giving them a quick read, and maybe taking a technique or two out for a "test drive," you will clearly get the most out of this ACT SP/SR program by deeply engaging with the material and the practices provided. We suggest taking at least 2–3 hours for each module, and possibly more time if some of the experiential exercises expand to become a part of a daily personal practice. Furthermore, several of the modules directly ask you to devote time to daily practice over the course of a week or more and to reflect upon the sum of that work in your SR questions or group discussions.

Chapter 4 is designed to help those of you who wish to facilitate ACT SP/SR groups. As such, much of this chapter might be less relevant for the solo practitioner or group member. Consider this an "optional" chapter, unless you are thinking about bringing together a group as a facilitator. If you are planning to organize and facilitate a group, the chapter walks you through the steps needed to get a group together and helps you anticipate some of the ups and downs you might run into as the group proceeds.

The second part of the book walks you through a series of modules that provide experiential SP exercises and a series of SR questions. These practices are organized around the psychological flexibility model and they provide an opportunity for you to cultivate specific capacities. Training the mind in psychological flexibility has broad empirical support throughout several scalable levels of intervention (Hooper & Larsson, 2015; Powers et al., 2009; Ruiz, 2010). Our aim is to provide you with an opportunity to use ACT SP/SR to develop evidence-supported processes leading to personal transformation. As a result, most of this workbook does not follow the format of a technical manual or narrative journey. The second section of this book is a "hands-on" guide for your own ACT SP/SR journey.

We wish you well on this shared path of personal and professional growth. As we become available to our own mindfulness, compassion, and wisdom, we are better able to share these resources with those who suffer. A path like this requires self-direction, discipline, and dedication. We wish all of these for you, as well as an openness to the help available through our communities of clinicians and fellow travelers. We are all in this together, and the prevention and alleviation of human suffering is a cause worth dedicating ourselves to with an open heart and determined commitment.

Note: The contextual behavioral science (CBS) community appreciates that gender involves behaviors that can be viewed as a performative spectrum, and that the arbitrary application of binary gender constructs can be limiting and even stigmatizing to many. As a result, we have chosen to use the singular "they" pronoun wherever possible throughout this text. This flexibility in our working with the fluid rules of grammar and style, in response to context, is consistent with the psychological flexibility model and our aims in CBS. We hope this will work for all our readers, and thank you for coming along for the ride.

CHAPTER 2

The Conceptual Framework

The Core Elements of ACT SP/SR

The ACT model is an inherently experiential model, and as ACT therapists, we don't merely wish to "tell" clients information or help them to "restructure" their thoughts through therapy homework. As we will explore together, the ACT therapist seeks to create the context for experiential learning and the training of specific processes in the present moment and in the consultation room. We will learn about all of these processes, through working with ourselves. Through ACT SP/SR, we cultivate our own psychological flexibility and a deeper, holistic understanding and embodiment of the psychological change model we practice and share.

There are many possible reasons that we might choose to become clinicians, and each of us has a unique personal history of engagement with psychological problems that has contributed to our motivation to help others deal with life's challenges. While the variations on the theme are infinite, in some sense, we all enter into the profession drawn by personal awareness of human suffering and the intention of being of service to our fellow humans. ACT SP/SR involves deliberately engaging with your own suffering, using the same processes and techniques that you would commonly direct toward your clients. In this way, we can encounter our capacity for mindfulness, acceptance, and compassion and learn to direct the flow of these essential elements inward. This potentially allows us to take our experience of the therapy to a deeper place than the typical course of our education. Nevertheless, the commitment involved in pursuing a course of SP/SR might seem demanding, and we might not see the value of this approach to our development at first. We can just read some of the key texts and attend a couple of workshops given by identified trainers to grasp the principles, can't we? If we follow published ACT protocols with adherence, won't we be effective as ACT therapists? We feel so busy sometimes and overwhelmed by the systems in which we work—why should we invest time and focus into SP/SR?

In order to appreciate the rewards of an ACT SP/SR approach, let's explore the principles involved in the learning and application of ACT and define some of the qualities that we are looking to develop as ACT therapists. As we begin our ACT SP/SR program, it is important to understand the specific value of personal practice for ACT therapists and to appreciate the science supporting this course of study. While many approaches to ACT might invite the therapist to look within as a part of learning the therapy, ACT SP/SR offers a unique contribution to the ACT therapist's personal and professional development, leading to being better equipped to make a real difference in our clinical endeavors.

While all approaches to therapy require a competent therapist to be grounded in the underlying theoretical assumptions of the model, ACT is unique in the breadth and scope of its conceptual basis. Emerging, as it does, from the behavior analytic tradition, ACT uses the term *behavior* to refer to every and any action that an organism can take. Daydreaming, jumping, designing an atom bomb, remembering, or baking a cake are all defined as "behavior" in the ACT literature and in this book, too. This is very important because ACT is based on the idea that we can apply the same scientific rules and principles to our understanding of mental behaviors that we apply to the learning of observable behaviors (Hayes et al., 1999).

As we will discuss, ACT is grounded in a particular philosophy of science, which suggests a specific approach to the analysis of human behavior. Upon this philosophical basis, the foundations of ACT expand to include a specific theory of language and cognition that informs the form and function of the therapy itself (Hayes et al., 1999). Rather than being an abstract set of ideas, this theoretical approach to thinking and verbal behavior is supported by a global and ongoing research initiative. In turn, this basic research is supported by applied research that seeks to test which processes are active in ACT and how we might achieve our best psychotherapeutic outcomes.

Thankfully, we don't need to be an expert in every level of theory that supports an ACT intervention in order to do good therapy. However, a deeper understanding of the building blocks of the therapy can help us to apply our techniques and relational strategies more flexibly and effectively. The ACT SP/SR approach seeks to help us develop an appreciation of these concepts through experiential learning, familiarizing ourselves with these processes in action as we notice them within ourselves. In turn, ACT therapists can develop the ability to apply this understanding in clinical settings in a way that is responsive to the client. Beyond technical and scientific elements, our SP/SR approach seeks to help us develop fundamental interpersonal skills, such as relationship building, collaboration, and active listening, which are also essential. Together, we explore and highlight specific components of an ACT therapeutic stance, including compassion, active empathy, and the shared experience of our common humanity.

Contextual Behavioral Science

Taking a closer look at the core elements of ACT, we find the therapy situated within a branch of psychology known as contextual behavioral science (CBS). CBS is a recently developed yet exponentially growing movement within psychology, which has been described as a "broad church" that encompasses three primary areas of knowledge development (Foody et al., 2014): a philosophy of science, a basic science theory of cognition and language, and a group of applied psychological interventions and psychotherapies.

The Philosophical Base: Functional Contextualism

Philosophy of science is emphasized in ACT because our philosophical assumptions have important consequences. For example, these assumptions can impact how we approach significant clinical issues, such as the relative value of questioning the truth versus falsehood of our clients' negative beliefs about themselves. All clinicians and scientists have philosophical assumptions, but many have never consciously articulated these assumptions. Absence of clarity regarding our philosophical approach can prevent us from a direct examination of the consequences of our philosophy. Furthermore, most of us did not arrive at our assumptions through deliberate philosophical analysis regarding the act of psychotherapy. We may have simply proceeded by approaching psychological science with the implicit assumptions that we have derived from our learning histories. In such cases, we begin without really thinking through where we stand. Our perspective may be less than deliberate, so *something is lost*.

It is likely that many clinicians begin to "do ACT" by simply adding ACT-derived techniques or mindfulness practices to their existing approach. While this may add something of value to the work, there is so much more that can be gained by a comprehensive study of the whole ACT approach. By encountering and internalizing a functional contextualist philosophical stance, we can change the entire frame of the psychotherapy relationship in powerful ways. Toward this end, we provide a brief introduction to our philosophy of science, with an examination of the *functional* and *contextual* elements separately. Following this introduction to functional contextualism, we provide a few reflective questions that link this perspective to your clinical work with your clients and yourself.

The best way for us to convey the meaning of *functional* in the approach is by way of example. Imagine a rat that is involved in behavioral research. This rat is found in an "operant chamber," a common tool in basic behavioral research that typically contains levers, lights, and a food or water dish. For this example, you have only to picture a chamber with a single lever. There are many ways a rat in a chamber can push the lever: with its nose, its left paw, its right paw, or its butt. One of us (Trent) used to work in a behavioral pharmacology lab and once witnessed a rat climb to the top of the chamber and then allow its body to fall on top of the lever. Many other possibilities exist. Most persons in the mental health professions think structurally and, as such, they would view all of these different lever-pressing behaviors as fundamentally different because the form or structure of each behavior is different. However, the functional contextualist *would view those responses in terms of function rather than structure*—that is, they would view those responses as identical because the function (i.e., the purpose) is the same: to push the lever. The form or "topography" (i.e., structure) of the behavior is not as useful for doing behavioral science and is thus a needless distraction.

In contrast, the *Diagnostic and Statistical Manual of Mental Disorders* (DSM) system is derived from a structural way of thinking about clinical problems. Anxiety disorders provide a useful example. The criteria set for each disorder within this category defines the disorder based on its form. For example, panic disorder involves fear of physical sensations. Simple phobias involve a fear of a specific object, activity, or situation. Generalized anxiety disorder is defined based on chronic worry about many different things. But each of these disorders is the same functionally: they function to avoid or escape anxiety-eliciting stimuli. In fact, we can extend the example even further to include most forms of psychopathology and still observe a shared functional class of behavior: experiential avoidance. Furthermore, even in those cases where a biological etiology is primary, there are likely experiential avoidance functions present that exacerbate the difficulty. Schizophrenia provides an example of this kind. The psychotic symptoms have a presumed biological etiology, but it's not uncommon for a person with schizophrenia to try to "run" from their voices, for example. This frequently has the consequence of increasing their experience of those symptoms while narrowing their repertoire in the presence of them. "Experiential avoidance" refers to any behavior that functions to avoid or escape aversive private experiences, including thoughts and feelings.

Contextualism, the second part of the term *functional contextualism*, reminds us that this is a pragmatic philosophy of science that focuses on the "act in context." In this approach, the "unit of analysis" is the behavior of a whole organism in context. This means that the entire context surrounding such a behavior, rather than its individual elements, is of interest. Functional contextualism chooses to focus on the prediction and influence of the act in context, with necessary and sufficient precision, depth, and scope. The breadth of the context carved out for a given evaluation depends entirely on the usefulness of the boundary conditions, based on one's analytic goals.

Rather than seeking "absolute truths" by seeing how much our predictions accord with the building blocks of a conceptualized "external reality," functional contextualism involves a specific benchmark for determining the truth of any given scientific analysis. That benchmark criterion is known as "successful working." To put this colloquially means asking the question "Did it work at accomplishing the goals that I specified?" One must always verbally state what the desired end is and then evaluate items based on whether they produce the desired end. In this way, the truth criterion for an ACT-consistent analysis, specifically, is not whether a description is mapping or describing an event in an objective, external world, but rather whether the prediction or influence of behavior in the analysis "works."

Accordingly, at the conceptual bedrock of ACT, we find a decision that every aspect of this approach to science will be grounded in this functional contextualist perspective, with an ensuing specific set of assumptions. In practical and applied terms during psychotherapy, the principles of functional contextualism include an emphasis of the *function* of a behavior in context over the *form* of the behavior in question.

A therapist grounded in this philosophy will likely be more interested in influencing how negative thoughts affect a client's actions than in *changing the form or content of an individual's reported automatic thoughts.* For example, an ACT therapist operating from these functional contextual assumptions would be reluctant to engage in a debate with a client looking for the "evidence for" and the "evidence against" her belief that she was a "bad mother." Instead, the ACT therapist would be more interested in creating the conditions where this mother could learn to notice herself thinking "I am a bad mother," while she reliably acted in ways that were her heart's deepest desire for how she would wish to parent. The therapist would seek to create a context in which this client could experience herself having a thought, but not basing her behavior upon what that thought says. The therapist would not attempt to change or suppress the thought "I am a bad mother" directly, but would rather create contingencies where the client could change her behaviors and act in ways that were personally meaningful, even when such a thought might arise. In this way, our relationship to our mental events and our direct engagement with valued actions become more important than the mental events themselves. As you might expect, there are further, more detailed parameters that make up the whole of this philosophical approach. However, holding these foundational functional contextualist principles in mind can deeply influence the way you learn and practice ACT SP/SR.

Reflect upon the questions below and write an answer in the space provided. We hope that pausing to reflect on the value of deepening your appreciation of a functional contextualist approach will empower your engagement with an ACT SP/SR approach.

Self-Reflective Questions

Can you imagine or remember an experience with a client when you, together, stressed the importance of understanding the function of their thinking over the client changing the form of their thoughts? If so, describe what your experience was like when you emphasized function over form.

_____

_____

_____

_____

_____

_____

_____

_____

Recall a time in your work when you and your client put their pursuit of valued behavioral aims first, rather than spending a lot of time challenging the validity of their negative thoughts. What did emphasizing behavior change and movement toward meaning, purpose, and vitality mean to you, as a therapist?

_____

_____

_____

_____

_____

_____

_____

_____

_____

_____

_____

_____

_____

Functional contextualism suggests that we view every behavior in its context and try to understand how an individual's learning history and current situation are exerting powerful influences on how they think, feel, and act. Furthermore, our responsibility as a therapist involves helping our clients to change their behaviors in meaningful ways through establishing a new relationship to their mental events. If you accept this view and this responsibility, what would it mean to you, as a psychotherapist? What would it mean to you as a person?

It makes me feel better equipped to help the client with effective tools. I feel it will evoke change that will stick.

I will feel more competent + confident as a clinician.

If you apply the principles of functional contextualism to your own life and address your own problems in a pragmatic way that emphasizes workability, what might be different for you?

I won't be as stressed worried, + perseverate. I will feel more at ease + better equipped to handle stressors

_____

_____

_____

_____

_____

_____

_____

_____

_____

The Theory of Cognition and Language: Relational Frame Theory

Relational frame theory (RFT) is a scientific theory of language and cognition that is grounded in functional contextualist assumptions and emerges from the behavior analytic tradition (Hayes, Barnes-Holmes, & Roche, 2001). RFT seeks to delineate and study human thinking and verbal behavior in terms of the experimental science of learning. As such, RFT serves as a conceptual framework, involving new models and concepts that provide useful ways of approaching the complexities of human verbal behavior.

Therapists may be better able to apprehend and apply ACT techniques when they understand what RFT has to tell us about thinking, just as jazz musicians will be better able to improvise and play in harmony when they understand the underlying music theory, chord changes, and scales that are involved. RFT posits that our evolved capacity to derive relations between stimuli we perceive has led to our capacity for cognition and language. Just as functional contextualism forms a foundation for RFT, in turn, RFT is connected to the cognitive interventions involved in ACT.

In simple terms, RFT suggests that, at its core, language involves the process of mentally relating events to one another. Furthermore, this process of relating events can also transform somatic, sensory, and behavioral functions. Our ability to derive relations among stimuli has likely provided a tremendous advantage for our human species. It's advantageous because it affords a substantial economy of learning, allowing us to relate events without explicit training. Furthermore, we can respond to verbal or cognitive rules about contingencies without needing to be exposed to the contingencies themselves. For example, I can be told, "Don't touch the hot stove, you will burn your fingers and need to go to the hospital." When I hear this, I can imagine the pain of the burned fingers and base my subsequent behavior on that cognitive rule. I don't need to actually burn my fingers in order to learn. Imagine what an advantage this kind of learning is for an entire species. Language obviously also allows humans to cooperate at a phenomenal level. We humans are a super-cooperative species, and RFT as applied to evolutionary science suggests that this cooperation may be our chief evolutionary advantage (Hayes & Long, 2013).

From an RFT perspective, cognition and language are described as "derived relational responding" or "relational framing." Relational framing involves three specific features: mutual entailment, combinatorial entailment, and transformation of stimulus function.

Mutual entailment involves a "bidirectional" learning process. For example, learning that the word *ball* represents an actual, physical ball, we readily derive the relation in the other direction. This means that we derive, without any explicit training, that an actual ball is "the same" as the word *ball*. After learning these relations, a child can see a novel ball and still name it with the word *ball*, even though this specific naming behavior has not been trained. *Combinatorial entailment* occurs when mutually entailed relations combine. For example, if one learns that *ball* is the same as an actual ball, and also that the Polish word *piłka* is the same as an actual ball, one will derive, without any specific training, that *piłka* and *ball* are the same. *Transformation of stimulus functions* refers to the functions of one stimulus transforming those of another. Continuing with the example of an actual ball and the words *piłka* and *ball*, consider a situation in which an individual had an aversive experience with a ball. Perhaps the person played baseball when younger and during a game was struck in the head by a pitched or batted ball. Because of this experience, baseballs came to elicit fear in the person. Prior to life training that fear, the word *ball* did not have a function, but now the word *ball* elicits a similar fear response to seeing a physical ball. If this person is a native-English speaker who learns to speak Polish, upon learning the word *piłka*, that word would also begin to have the function of triggering an aversive response. A word that had previously been neutral now elicits a fear response, reflecting a transformation of the function of the word.

Several clinical implications can be derived from the RFT account of human language and cognition. First, learning, including relational learning, is additive, not subtractive—that is, new relations are constantly being learned and old relations cannot be erased. This suggests that clinical interventions that attempt to "delete" old learning cannot work and, in fact, just add new learning to a person's relational repertoire. For example, if I attempt to use "thought stopping" to help a person with obsessive–compulsive disorder (OCD) cease having intrusive thoughts, I am likely to increase the frequency and intensity of their OCD symptoms. We can help clients to elaborate and adapt their relational networks and learn new ways of thinking and being. However, we can't really teach them to "unlearn" old relations. While occasionally new learning can be so superimposed over older responses such that it seems to suppress earlier learning, we can't delete our previous histories, and the older repertoires can reemerge under certain conditions. Attempts at avoidance and suppression of mental events are doomed to failure at best, and backfiring at worst.

Second, relational framing evolved because it helped humans survive, and did so partly because a core feature is that it gets us to interact with words as if they are literally real. This can be useful when we are busy solving problems in the external environment, but it can also lead to a number of unnecessary emotional struggles. RFT helps us understand these processes and implies helpful interventions. Relational learning can come to dominate other factors that regulate behavior, such as direct experience of environmental contingencies. This is observed when clients continue to engage in unworkable activity despite receiving environmental feedback countless times.

Imagine you are working with a psychotherapy client who is a female graduate student. In her personal history, she has learned the verbal rule "If I speak in public, I may freeze up with fear and embarrass myself. I'll fail as a public speaker." That fear might cause the client to avoid public speaking, even when it harms her academic or professional career. The more this client aims to stop thinking these thoughts, or suppress them from arising, the more likely it is that these thoughts will emerge with greater frequency and intensity. The entire affair of public speaking might become intensely aversive. Even if this person is stuck in situations where she needs to speak in public, and even if she does a great job, with many people praising her performance, the verbal behaviors of self-condemnation and predicting failures may persist and she may continue to fear and dread public speaking. An ACT-consistent intervention, grounded in RFT, would aim to help establish a context where this client could come to experience the mental event of thinking "I'll fail as a public speaker" in such a way that facilitates a transformation of stimulus function. For example, the client might use a mindfulness practice, repeating the phrase "I'll fail as a public speaker" like a mantra, until its stimulus functions began to change. The client and therapist might have the client repeat the phrase for a few minutes, and then make a video recording of her delivering a brief public talk. Together, they would both witness how the client could, in fact, engage in her valued action, even in the presence of an intrusive and threatening series of thoughts. While this example of an ACT-consistent intervention might seem similar in form to exposure or behavioral experiments from CBT—"disproving" the negative thought through action and "desensitizing" the client to fear through exposure—the proposed function of the intervention is very different. The ACT therapist is not aiming to change any cognitions directly or to reduce the intensity or form of any emotional response. The aim here is to create a context wherein the client's internal verbalizations exert a different function, allowing the client to persist in a valued action, even in the presence of difficult internal events. The intervention is hypothesized as taking place "outside" the client in the manipulation of the context, rather than "inside" the client in the hypothetical change of thoughts and feelings directly.

Reflect upon the questions below and write an answer in the space provided. Let's consider the ways that understanding RFT might improve your ability to work with ACT-consistent moves with your clients and with yourself.

Self-Reflective Questions

RFT suggests that one of the core processes that fuels psychotherapy progress involves the transformation of stimulus function of mental events, meaning that gradually we might experience the same mental event, but that it will exert a very different influence upon our thoughts, feelings, and behaviors. Can you recall a time your relationship to a mental event, memory, or distressing thought changed dramatically? Can you recall a time when the way you were affected by a troubling inner experience transformed so that some of your struggle and suffering changed? If so, describe this below:

Yes - related to public speaking fears.

When you experienced a transformation of how certain mental events affected you, what did this mean for your state of mind, your possible behaviors, and your freedom of action in your life?

I felt calmer & less anxious

_____

_____

_____

_____

_____

_____

_____

_____

_____

_____

When you experienced a "transformation of stimulus function," did this come about through greater acceptance, mindful awareness, and deeper engagement in taking meaningful action in your life? If not, what else was happening for you?

Yes it did — all 3. Had to accept
doing presentations, was more mindful
of the act + that I could do it + not
be perfect; I actually started to not
mind doing presentations + felt more confident.

_____

_____

_____

_____

_____

_____

_____

How can you imagine that an understanding of RFT principles and a lived experience of the dynamics of relational responding can empower your psychotherapy further?

By imparting the skills for cl usage.

CBS Psychotherapies and Applications: "ACT & Co."

ACT is an empirically tested clinical approach, designed to improve psychological health and well-being (Hayes et al., 2012) that is grounded in CBS, functional contextualism, and RFT. ACT has evolved from the behavior analytic tradition, CBT, humanistic therapies, existential approaches to psychology, evolution science, and Eastern philosophy. At this point, over 200 RCTs and thousands of peer-reviewed studies have supported the utility and efficacy of ACT processes and procedures (*https://contextualscience.org/state_of_ the_act_evidence*). While ACT is the most popular and best studied CBS intervention, there are several other applications and interventions that are growing within the CBS community. Functional analytic psychotherapy (Tsai, Kohlenberg, Kanter, Holman, & Loudon, 2012), compassion-focused therapy (CFT; Gilbert, 2010; Tirch, Schoendorff, & Silberstein, 2014), the DNA-V model (Hayes & Ciarrochi, 2015), clinical RFT (Villatte, Villatte, & Hayes, 2015), PROSOCIAL group development (*www.prosocial.world*), and a range of other rapidly developing technologies have a relationship to CBS and are, to varying degrees, outgrowths of the CBS community's mission. In this book, we focus on ACT from an SP/SR approach. However, SP/SR has been applied to other contextual science-related psychotherapies, such as CFT (Kolts, Bell, Bennett-Levy, & Irons, 2018) and other cognitive and behavioral approaches, such as schema therapy (Farrell & Shaw, 2018) and CBT (Bennett-Levy et al., 2015). Workbooks on some of these approaches are available in this Guilford series, Self-Practice/Self-Reflection Guides for Psychotherapists.

ACT has developed over the past 35 years through a distinctively systematic and stepwise process. Years before ACT ever emerged as a psychotherapy, the original ACT developers first constructed the philosophical basis for the approach (Hayes, 1993). This philosophy of science, in turn, led to RFT, which formed the basis of ACT as a form of treatment. The three levels of CBS (philosophy of science, basic theory of cognition, and therapeutic application) represent an intentional approach to develop a science focused on the alleviation of human suffering that is grounded in evidence-based processes from the ground up. A competent ACT clinician will typically aim to have some degree of understanding of these three domains of CBS, each of which presents unique conceptual challenges and opportunities. Importantly, recognized and peer-reviewed ACT trainers are expected to be conversant in all of these areas, and the process of peer review reflects this. For our purposes, SP/SR allows us to explore the connection that ACT establishes to its theoretical underpinnings from the ground up. Each element of ACT represents ways of knowing and approaching human behavior, which can be developed through personal practice and experience.

Building upon the Foundations of ACT: A Closer Look at RFT

As we focus on the application of the ACT clinical model from the viewpoint of SP/SR, we endeavor to avoid using technical terms. Indeed, unfavorable ACT client feedback is often associated with the therapy being too technique focused, or wrapped up in conceptual complexity (Brock, Batten, Walser, & Robb, 2015). As you have likely already noticed or already know, RFT is so steeped in technical language and behavior analytic assumptions that we run the risk of being balanced too heavily toward the technical as opposed to lived processes if we get too wrapped up in the conceptual. However, as we proceed, we wish you to be able to *absorb and embody* some of the key therapeutic moves and realizations that emerge from this way of understanding human cognition.

There is debate, in fact, as to whether one needs to learn RFT *at all* in order to become an effective ACT practitioner, and it may be unlikely that you would converse with the client using RFT terms. However, *having an understanding of this foundation can deepen your approach*. For example, if we imagined that you were choosing clothing suitable for travel to a hotter climate, you wouldn't need to be an expert in the laws of physics, such as the mathematics involved in heat exchange, in order to go shopping. However, it would be useful to know that we tend to feel cooler in clothes made of linen fabric than those made of heavy wool, as linen promotes more "breathability" when placed against a human body. You need to know enough to get the job done, and sometimes deepening your knowledge can even deepen your understanding and practice.

"Deriving Me Crazy": RFT Concepts as Clinical Building Blocks

We expect that our readers have a range of familiarity with behavior analytic terms. Wherever you are on that continuum, it can be helpful to come back to an orientation to what some of our most basic terms actually mean. For example, that a "stimulus" actually refers to an event or quality that surrounds a behavior, rather than a particular "thing." In essence, a *stimulus* is a term that represents a change in our environment, and that means any change at all. In practice, this translates to our experience of noticing just about anything that happens around us. If the lights turn on in your apartment, then we can call that a stimulus. If you just heard your dog barking in the yard, we can call that a stimulus. Holding a coin in your hand and noticing its size and design can be a stimulus, too. When we learn something about one stimulus and then we learn something else about another stimulus, and we experience these stimuli in relation to each other, our minds automatically derive a relation between the two. As it turns out, these relations lead to more than the sum of their parts and create the spark we need for our consciousness to unfold.

Let's use the example of coins as a stimuli, in a classic ACT example of how we derive relations between stimuli. Imagine that you were entirely new to the currency in the United Kingdom, and we were introducing it to you. If I were to show you that the 20-pence (20p) coin was smaller than the 1-pound (£1) coin, and that the £1 coin was, in turn, smaller than the 50-pence (50p) coin, what could you tell me about the relationship between the 20p coin and the 50p coin? You might say that the 20p coin is smaller than the 50p coin, or that the 50p coin is bigger than the 20p coin. Both of these statements would be entirely correct. However, I didn't tell you that—you simply "worked it out for yourself." In RFT language, we would say that you *derived* that relationship, a relationship based on the relative size of the coins.

What if I asked you which coin was better, or which coin had more value? If I showed you all three coins, but only *directly* trained you to know that the £1 coin had more value than the 50p coin, and that the 20p coin had less value than the 50p coin, you could, seemingly automatically, *derive* the knowledge that the 20p coin was worth less than the £1 coin.

This process of deriving relations can be so obvious to us, and so ingrained, that it can seem nearly absurd when we first encounter this example in ACT or RFT training. Deriving relations is something that we humans do all the time; it is foundational to the process of thinking and an activity that distinguishes us from other creatures. Derived relational responding develops early in our lives and is elaborated through years of training in our human social interactions. For example, if as a child a parent offered you a bunch of coins and asked you to choose one for yourself, it is likely that you will pick the biggest coin. As your learning develops and you become familiar with the value or worth of coins and you realize that a £1 coin can buy you twice as many sweets as a 50p coin, then you might pick a different coin.

Rather than thinking of *derived relational responding* as a separate process from thinking, we invite you to consider this term as a description of the very fabric of all mental activity. By describing the act of cognition in terms of its basic functional units, RFT researchers and CBS practitioners are better able to frame scientific questions and experiments that can predict and influence our mental activity with precision, depth, and scope. In this way, we have an appreciation of the finely grained dynamics of human thought that is built into the design of the ACT SP/SR method, as well as all ACT interventions. If we can better understand the ways in which we respond to mental events, and the manner in which these mental events can contribute to our suffering, we have the opportunity to take action to alter the excessive influence of unhelpful thoughts, or those inner experiences that lead us to respond in narrow and inflexible ways.

In this way, we might devise methods to change, or transform, the function that a stimulus event will have in influencing our actions and experience. As we discussed, the *transformation of stimulus functions* is essential to the aims of ACT therapists when they are working with their clients, or even when they are turning the focus of their ACT approach inward through SP/SR training. Let's look at another simple example of this process in action. To begin, let's remember the experience of eating a light and fluffy omelet, perfectly prepared. Perhaps you have had a vegetable omelet with fresh vegetables, or one with beautifully creamy and sharp Swiss cheese. The stimulus function of remembering that omelet for many would be a pleasant memory of sensation, or a signal to the stomach to release gastric juices in preparation for a good meal. For many, just the idea of a tasty omelet will provoke a little hunger or pleasant mental events, and these mental events will exert an influence on our bodies and our behavioral urges.

Now imagine that you have cracked an egg to make just such a delicious omelet, and when the egg dropped into the frying pan, you noticed that it had considerably gone bad. What comes to mind as you consider this? Are you noticing what this rotten egg would have looked like, or are you noticing the revolting sulfur smell that this egg would have given off? Can you imagine cooking this egg and putting it in an omelet to eat? Perhaps even the idea of this triggers some nausea or a general sense of disgust. As our teaching story has changed, the stimulus function of the word *egg* or *omelet* has shifted from something that triggers hunger to something that might even trigger nausea. In the simplest of ways, *the function of the stimulus has transformed* with just a few words communicated from one person to another through written language. Understanding-derived relational responding can help us to understand how *changing the context in which we experience a stimulus might result in transformation of stimulus function.*

Additionally, thinking in terms of how we humans persistently derive new relations among stimuli can help us understand how the functions of one stimulus might be *transferred* to other stimuli. This helps us understand how our experience of one context or memory might affect our behavior in other situations in the future. Of course, we can expect that a youth who has experienced bullying by a group of students at school might experience anxiety when seeing any group of young people together. This child might come to avoid going to school or youth clubs, and may even feel anxiety later in life in social situations that involved group gatherings. We could imagine how a survivor of a road traffic accident might feel sick when smelling gasoline and avoid driving. These examples of the *transfer of stimulus function*, and specifically the behavioral avoidance that can develop across time and situation, are all better understood when we understand the basic building blocks of how we think and develop relational networks in the mind.

In this way, RFT can help us to understand how relationships are derived between events, internal or external, and the subsequent impact on behavioral choices.

From RFT in Concept to ACT in Action

Deriving of stimulus relations, transfer of stimulus functions, and the transformation of stimulus functions represent some of the fundamental building blocks of mental functioning throughout the lifespan. ACT interventions create powerful contexts and relevant learning experiences that can intentionally facilitate the transformation of stimulus functions, leading to an enhancement in flexible and effective responding to challenging situations and greater movement toward lives of meaning, purpose, and vitality. In a psychotherapy context, these processes are facilitated through the therapeutic alliance. In our ACT SP/SR work, we seek to create a powerful context of mindfulness, acceptance, and self-compassion that can facilitate an enhancement of psychological flexibility and the capacity to respond more effectively as a psychotherapist and fully engaged human.

The Problem of Experiential Avoidance

ACT was developed from early research on the impact of experiential avoidance on behavioral disorders (Hayes et al., 1996). As several decades of research have demonstrated, persistent attempts to avoid our internal experiences lead to an intensification of psychological suffering and underpin many apparent psychological disorders (Chawla & Ostafin, 2007; Hayes, Wilson, Gifford, Follette, & Strosahl, 1996). As a result, ACT interventions often target a client's patterns of avoidance. However, we should be mindful that not all experiential avoidance or attempts to overtly control our cognitions are inherently wrong moves. For example, if we were triggered into intense anger during an important meeting at work with our job on the line, we might choose to distract ourselves and carry on as calmly as possible, rather than risk an explosive argument with our supervisor. Bonanno, Papa, Lalande, Westphal, and Coifman (2004) demonstrated in their research that the suppression of emotional expression in certain contexts can be beneficial, and they suggest that moving toward expressive flexibility with a sensitivity to contingencies is often beneficial.

Of course, avoiding actual threats and painful experiences in the outside world can be necessary and useful. For instance, when we are hiking on the Appalachian Trail, "avoiding" a bear is probably a very good idea. One of the reasons that we try to apply a strategy of avoidance so often to our mental experiences is that avoidance is so essential to our survival in terms of our interactions with our environment. Predators, contaminants, natural disasters, heights, and a host of other threats must be avoided if we are to survive. Unfortunately for us, when we apply that same strategy to our mental experiences, things tend to go badly for us. The more we attempt to avoid having certain thoughts, emotions, and memories, the more they show up. So, in ACT SP/SR, we aim to explore and understand our patterns of inner avoidance and to cultivate our capacity to bring a gentle and self-compassionate acceptance to our experience of the present moment, and all that it contains.

To understand the significance and subsequent targeting of experiential avoidance from an ACT perspective, let's look at the example of a young mother who has been diagnosed with postpartum OCD and who is unwilling to bathe her infant. Given terrifying obsessional thoughts, the mother experiences severe anxiety when imagining bathing her first child. Her mind generates spontaneous images of drowning her baby. These thoughts horrify her, and she automatically tries to suppress and avoid the thoughts. As we would expect, this only results in the thoughts showing up more and more often, and often with greater intensity. Thanks to our capacity to respond to imaginal events as if they were real, these images cause the mother to have an accelerated threat response, with great ensuing shame and anxiety. The mother might experience associated cognitions, such as "Only a bad parent would think such thoughts" and therefore "I am a bad parent," and she would experience these mental events as very real and terribly distressing. Her patterns of internal experiential avoidance result in an amplification of her suffering. In time, the mother's avoidance of internal events expands and she begins to avoid bathing her infant entirely, depending on her own relatives and spouse to help out. In this case, experiential avoidance has grown from the internal realm into outside behaviors. In this way, the woman's suffering has not only been exacerbated by the amplification of painful thoughts and emotions but the quality of her life and her possibilities of living her values have been diminished by the constriction of her actions through avoidance and overcontrol.

From an ACT-consistent perspective we view the entire example in terms of the functional analysis of the contingencies involved in shaping and maintaining the woman's behaviors. It is not simply the *form* of her negative thoughts and anxiety that we are most interested in and seek to target but the *function* of those private events. In some schools of CBT, we would seek to elicit the negative automatic thoughts that this woman was experiencing, and we would train her to directly challenge and dispute these thoughts. ACT seeks a different course, in which we don't begin by aiming to change the form of her thinking directly. We would first seek to draw out and clarify the patterns of avoidance that characterize the woman's pattern of relating to such thoughts. We would help this new mother to develop a new relationship to these thoughts, where she could recognize them as mental events, rather than real events in the world. She would practice a new way of being with this troubling mental material, learning to hold these experiences lightly and with self-kindness. She would aim to clarify the valued actions that she could choose to engage in despite her mind weaving terrible and shameful images. The context of a supportive and compassionate therapeutic alliance would serve as the foundation for building a new experience of her troubling thoughts and feelings. From an ACT perspective, "a primary source of psychopathology (as well as a process exacerbating the impact of other sources of psychopathology) is the way that language and cognition interact with direct contingencies to produce an inability to persist or change behavior in the service of long-term valued ends" (Hayes et al., 2006, p. 6). As such, the desired outcome of ACT is not the reduction of the frequency or intensity of discomfiting private events but the increasing willingness to experience discomfort, be more present to direct contingencies, and choose behaviors aligned to valued directions (Hayes et al., 2012).

The ACT Therapeutic Stance

Empathy and warmth (Rogers, 1951) are central to the therapeutic stance taken in ACT, and genuineness is pivotal to client engagement in the therapeutic relationship. These elements share common ground with most effective psychotherapeutic orientations (Norcross & Lambert, 2011). However, authenticity from an ACT perspective is a very specific and deeply held construct, underpinned by RFT. ACT therapy and ACT training begins with an appreciation of our common humanity and the universality of human suffering. In a highly collaborative and even vulnerable context, the ACT therapist adopts and sincerely conveys the notion to clients that we are all in the same boat (Bach & Moran, 2008). This speaks to the rewards and challenges facing prospective ACT therapists and to the opportunities provided by SP/SR. Through ACT SP/SR we aim to develop the ability to comprehend and utilize therapy technologies and techniques in a genuine and compassionate manner, for ourselves and for the clients we serve (Bennett-Levy et al., 2015).

The stance of the therapist in ACT is radical acceptance and respect for the client (Hayes et al., 1999). In this way, the ACT therapist models and embodies acceptance, psychological flexibility, and compassion, including compassion for oneself as a therapist. "Acceptance" in this context means acceptance of one's own experience and humanity in addition to acceptance of the client experience (Bach & Moran, 2008). This can be transmitted from therapist to client in many ways. For example, the therapist can model the tolerance of uncertainty and convey deep respect and nonjudgmental regard when experiencing silence and perhaps self-doubt in a clinical session. While practicing mindfulness, slowing the rate of respiration, and remaining intentionally emotionally open, the ACT therapist might say something like:

I am aware that we seem to have come to a pause. I notice my mind racing ahead suggesting a lot of things that I should do, but mostly I'm aware of wishing to be of genuine service to you in the here and now. So, I am wondering what is showing up for you as we sit together in this moment?

In this way, respect, compassion, and the intention of collaboration is clearly communicated.

As we will see, evidence-based processes involved in psychological flexibility—such as contacting the present moment, practicing willingness, and letting go of attachment to the literal meaning of thoughts—are all involved in this response. This response requires patience and courage. By virtue of the patient's own empathy and the activation of mirror neurons, the implicational level of this human interaction is experienced and internalized through the therapeutic relationship, moment by moment. This stands in contrast to what can happen when a therapist is less open and accepting of their own experience. Stepping outside of the ACT stance, gripped by a need to solve problems with urgency and anxiety, we can sometimes rush to fill the silence during "stuck moments" by diving into psychoeducation, producing new "worksheets," or filling the intersubjective space with a lot of therapist talking and pontification. This isn't as likely to move the active psychotherapeutic processes that we are targeting, in our clients or in ourselves. By contrast, modeling commitment and showing up to discomfort (willingness) facilitates both therapist and client maintaining a present-moment focus that affords a valuable learning opportunity that may have been lost.

Similarly, if a client returns to a session stating that "This therapy is really not working, I don't think you understand how bad it is for me," the ACT therapist might say something like:

It sounds like you feel misunderstood. I want to get closer to your frustration and to really appreciate it. Just now, I notice my mind suggesting that maybe I am a bad therapist or I am doing a poor job. But I'm not interested in getting hooked by that. In this moment, I am making room for that and focusing on you and what you need. It would mean a lot to me to understand your frustration more fully. Can you help me to understand how bad it is for you, in the moment, please? What is showing up for you, here and now?

In this way, again, present-moment focus is maintained, thus allowing new learning—but additionally, the therapist is modeling showing up to the experience, even if it is distressing, in the service of what matters to the therapist, with both client and therapist moving toward valued action in the face of distressing inner experiences.

In addition to genuineness being associated with positive client outcome (Rogers, 1957), therapist experiential avoidance and safety behaviors have been suggested to interfere with adherence to treatment models (Waller, 2009; Waller, Stringer, & Meyer, 2012). Accordingly, the therapist's awareness of the potential for their own avoidance is significant in adopting an ACT stance. Furthermore, it has been suggested that courage may be a significant component of moving toward a more valued life (Wetterneck, Lee, Smith, & Hart, 2013) and rather than acting defensively in the face of criticism, the therapist modeling courage may be beneficial. In adopting an ACT-consistent therapeutic stance, the therapist is also demonstrating attunement to fluctuations of affect and cognition on a moment-to-moment basis, for both themselves and the client. The ACT SP/SR approach seeks to help ACT therapists hone the mindfulness, self-compassion, and flexible responding they will need to be able to embody and realize this stance. This is particularly important for the ACT therapist and requires utilizing "reflection-in-action" (Schön, 1983) or, as described in the behavioral tradition, "tracking" behaviors and modifying our responses based on changing contingencies in real time. "Reflection-in-action"

(Schön, 1983) can take place during and after session, during personal practice, and in clinical supervision.

ACT SP/SR and the ACT Stance

The clinical training of ACT in the classroom has often consisted of a didactic approach (Georgescu & Brock, 2016) with further training available through workshops and conferences for graduate and postgraduate practitioners. Typically, academic centers utilize in-class role plays, case conferences, and clinical supervision in a mixed-methods approach. However, many clinicians who are adopting ACT practice now will have already been trained in graduate school in other approaches, sometimes several years ago. Many of the therapists seeking to practice it, or even currently practicing ACT, will never have had the opportunity to learn the therapy in a structured didactic or supervisory setting, let alone in graduate school. These clinicians will probably seek training through self-instruction via books, online resources, and journal articles. Such training can, and should, be augmented through private individual supervision, peer supervision, experiential workshops, and conference attendance. Adding experiential components to ACT training has been found to be beneficial (Hayes, 2004; Luoma & Vilardaga, 2013), particularly in terms of developing proficiency in practicing the active components of ACT, making connections between theory and professional practice, and improving the use of psychotherapy supervision (Batten & Santanello, 2009). Importantly, attending workshops alone is not necessarily enough to effectively become an ACT therapist.

Research has shown that a clinician's skill acquisition can remain low postworkshop, and that skill development requires consolidation through supervision and consultations (Walser, Karlin, Trockel, Mazina, & Taylor, 2013). In order to fully implement this powerful approach, a comprehensive path to mastery needs to be composed. Often, we are left to find our own way in this process. This can be a tricky path for busy clinicians and students, and finding a smooth course of professional education and growth in ACT requires a great deal of effort and commitment for most of us. Perhaps the key to maintaining an ACT therapeutic stance can be found in balancing: fidelity to the ACT treatment model; implementation of CBS philosophy and theory in practice; and an embodiment of mindfulness, acceptance, and compassion.

In all of this, modeling the wisdom of radical acceptance of self and other is central to ACT. Research has demonstrated that an SP/SR approach can help us to develop these precise competencies. In this way, ACT and SP/SR are perfectly complementary with each other and hold great promise in combination. Given the unevenness and complexity of access to consistent ACT training experiences globally, we suggest that personal practice in the form of SP/SR can make a significant contribution to ACT therapist development. Bennett-Levy and colleagues (2009) have suggested that while personal reading and access to lectures can be helpful in acquiring declarative, theoretical knowledge, these methods alone lead to limited gain with regard to the procedural use of specific skills in action. Role play and clinical demonstrations have been found to be beneficial in acquiring conceptual understanding and technical knowledge

(Bennett-Levy et al., 2009; Georgescu & Brock, 2016). However, in terms of developing interpersonal and reflective skills, Bennett-Levy and colleagues have shown that reflective practice and self-experiential learning offer a deeper way of moving from theory to practice for clinicians.

ACT SP/SR offers the opportunity to combine reflective practice and experiential learning, which affords the opportunity to achieve the balance of conceptualization/ technique and interpersonal flexibility more effectively. Utilizing SP/SR, as suggested in this workbook, facilitates opportunities to develop a deeper understanding of the philosophy and theory that underpins ACT; to become more cognizant of the components of ACT and ACT-consistent techniques; to develop personal qualities of courage, compassion, perspective taking, and psychological flexibility; and to thereby engage clinically at the process level in a genuine and authentic fashion that then allows a safe therapeutic space to be developed collaboratively with those clients we serve.

CHAPTER 3

Guidance for Participants

This chapter is necessary and important reading for anyone involved with ACT SP/SR. Facilitators, participants, supervisors, or anyone involved in the provision of an ACT SP/SR program will find the information provided here essential to an effective SP/SR program. Together, we review what to consider before beginning the program and how to set yourself up to get the most out of the experience.

The developers of SP/SR observed differences in how much individuals benefit from their experience in SP/SR. They then looked into what factors and behaviors differentiated those participants who experienced more benefit than others. They found that the level of engagement in the program is key to the benefit individuals experience (Bennett-Levy & Lee, 2014). Thus, we explore how to prepare for your ACT SP/SR program in the service of maximizing engagement, meeting your individual valued aims, and in turn, getting the most benefit you can out of your work. There are many benefits and desirable outcomes to experiencing ACT from the inside out. As mentioned, these include a more precise and in-depth understanding of ACT, enhanced self-awareness and reflection skills, expanded perspective taking, and a more psychologically flexible approach to therapy or in other areas of living.

This chapter is divided into three sections. First, we look at ACT SP/SR in different contexts—in a group, on your own, with a peer, or with a supervisor—and provide guidance for effectively working within these various contexts. Second, we explore the practicalities of SP/SR and how to navigate these in order to enhance engagement and reap the most benefit. These include how to choose your valued aims and areas of focus for the ACT SP/SR work, time requirements and management, when to start your program, and how to take good care of yourself throughout the process. Third, we focus on the key processes and capacities involved in self-reflection. In SP/SR it is assumed that everyone has different capabilities and available skills for reflection that vary through time and context. So, in this section, we include guidelines for cultivating your capacity for self-reflection.

ACT SP/SR in Different Contexts

ACT SP/SR can be conducted in a variety of different contexts and configurations. The following sections review important considerations for choosing which context to pursue. These contexts include self-guided ACT SP/SR or with others, such as ACT SP/SR with a peer, in groups, or with a supervisor.

Self-Guided ACT SP/SR

For many of us, there can be several reasons to choose self-guided SP/SR. Be it due to location, lack of contact with others in the profession, lack of access to necessary technology, personal preference, or other valued pursuits, you are the captain of your program. You are the one who will know what is best for you. However, it is wise to be aware of potential challenges that may arise when taking on a self-guided ACT SP/SR program. These challenges will vary from person to person and are based on individual differences. So, if you are choosing a self-guided program, it is important to consider your possible challenges in this approach. You may want to ask yourself:

- "Can I set aside regularly scheduled time to engage with the exercises?"
- "Can I independently develop clear aims for my program and track my progress?"
- "How can I keep myself motivated and engaged throughout the process?"
- "How will I cultivate and maintain my commitment?"

It is also important to remember that ACT SP/SR can unexpectedly evoke difficult or challenging emotional experiences and that developing a Personal Support Strategy prior to beginning the program is strongly suggested. Finally, we would like to remind you that, even if you choose self-guided ACT SP/SR, you are not alone. There are persons, both similar and different from you, working through these modules, and others in the Association for Contextual Behavioral Science (ACBS) community who are learning and living ACT. If you are interested in becoming more connected with individuals in the ACT SP/SR community, you can join our ACT SP/SR social media group on Facebook at *https://www.facebook.com/groups/actspsr*. If you are not already connected to fellow ACT practitioners, you can also join the larger ACT community by becoming a member of ACBS, connecting through their online resources, taking part in email discussion groups, or by attending local and international trainings and conferences (*www.contextualscience.org*). Additionally, simply remember that, in a sense, you are not alone in this work. No SP/SR program would be possible without those who have developed this model, those who have applied it, and those who have participated in and experienced it. So, if you are self-guiding your ACT SP/SR program, we invite you to remember that we are in this together, and unseen others are in it with you. Additional support or connection is available to you, if you communicate with the community.

Working on ACT SP/SR with Others

The creators and facilitators of SP/SR programs have consistent feedback from former participants that their experience was enhanced when shared with others (Bennett-Levy & Lee, 2014; Farrand, Perry, & Linsley, 2010). Working though the SP/SR modules with one or more persons and sharing the reflections with others can be a powerful and rewarding experience. This shared learning provides opportunities for deepening and expanding ACT SP/SR learning and creates a supportive, validating, and safe context for inner work and growth. All of this helps maintain engagement, stay on track, and accountability to personal commitments to the work. Whether you are working with one or more persons, it is helpful to consider the context in which you meet online, in person, or a combination of both. The following sections review the considerations to make for certain configurations of working through ACT SP/SR with others.

SP/SR with a Peer or Colleague

When choosing to work one-on-one with a peer or colleague, there are several suggested considerations. First, trust and confidentiality are of the utmost importance in SP/SR work with others. Is a high level of trust available in this relationship? Will confidentiality agreements be honored? Next, it is advised that you consider relative levels of experience, theoretical knowledge of ACT and CBS, and stages of clinical and professional development. Pairing up with someone who has a similar learning background and aims for the program helps maximize the experience for all involved. One final consideration for SP/SR work in pairs is how to ensure the time is shared equally between the two participants—both involved can take on this responsibility. You can monitor yourself to balance the time you spend listening and supporting the other and the time you use sharing and receiving support and encouragement from the person you are working with.

SP/SR in a Group

ACT SP/SR groups can take many forms and can be held in a variety of contexts. For example, groups can be held as a part of regular meetings for a team at a clinic or group practice. This kind of work is especially well suited as a part of peer supervision or in a university or other training program. The emphasis upon working with oneself with peer support is distinct from working in "group supervision" or "group therapy." In ACT SP/SR, we can give and receive support as equals sharing in the common humanity of human struggle. No one person will serve as the "therapist" or "problem solver" for any other. This can be humbling, and also can ground a group in an egalitarian and collaborative stance. This benefit, in and of itself, could recommend ACT SP/SR to peer-training contexts.

Given current communications technology, and the open and cooperative values of the CBS global community, there is literally a world of opportunity for you to find colleagues with whom you can share an ACT SP/SR experience. As mentioned earlier, groups can meet in person, online, or a combination of the two. Groups are encouraged to use online discussion forums, chat rooms, or interactive blogs or social media to create the right "space" for their ACT SP/SR work to flourish.

Newly forming ACT SP/SR groups should consider the aforementioned factors of trust and confidentiality. Certain contexts where participants work closely with one another, or where there are hierarchical or evaluative relationships at play, can inhibit a sense of safeness or willingness to engage in open disclosure and discourse. Beyond the subjective experience of safeness, certain disclosures and intimate discussions of personal struggles can affect professional relationships in practical ways, and all of this should be considered as a process of mutual consent and agreement in engaging in this kind of work. As we will discuss, an ACT SP/SR group should collaboratively address these factors and come to agreements of how to address issues of trust, safety, and confidentiality.

SP/SR with a Supervisor

ACT SP/SR can be a beneficial addition to the supervisory process. This can be done in a variety of forms and with an emphasis on various areas related to an individual's clinical training or supervision. As SP/SR work relates to development of both the personal self and the professional self, the guidance and care of a trusted supervisor can provide an appropriate and empowering environment while facing challenging material. Of course, given the personal nature of the work discussed, an awareness of interpersonal boundaries is paramount in such a context. Importantly, the supervisor should not shift into a therapist role, as the supervisee engages in ACT SP/SR. Rather, the supervision relationship can provide a reflective and safe context for trainees to work on themselves in the presence of another person. If you are working through your SP/SR program with a clinical supervisor, this can be done formally or in a more supportive fashion. The ACT SP/SR program and modules can become a regular part of the supervision meetings. The supervisor and supervisee can formally move though the modules in a targeted manner, similar to groups or SP/SR with a peer. Alternatively, supervision can provide needed support for individuals who completed more of a self-guided approach in tandem with supervision. In this more supportive approach, the supervisee can raise issues evoked by SP/SR in supervision as needed.

If SP/SR is being used more formally in supervision, there are many ways to tailor this program to meet the needs and aims of the supervisee. For example, with trainees less experienced with ACT, the modules can be used to enhance the participants' understanding and engagement with learning ACT processes and techniques. For those more experienced in ACT, the program can be individualized to focus on related therapeutic challenges, such as therapeutic relationship processes and therapists' own areas of psychological inflexibility, or can address any other personal struggles related to the clinical work being supervised.

Practicalities of SP/SR:
Maximizing Engagement and Reaping the Benefits

As psychotherapists, our attention is often focused on the aims of others, such as our clients, students, or trainees. In ACT SP/SR, *your* aims and intentions are the primary focus. This inward direction of awareness as a therapist may be a new and daunting experience at first. The process of selecting our own valued aims can also be an exciting and motivating experience. The SP/SR program provides guidance and support in clarifying those ACT SP/SR aims that are most important to you. We also provide guidance and practices for realizing those aims.

The ACT SP/SR program begins with a guided and experiential process to help you identify your own program's direction. There are a few things to consider when making this choice. Early on in the ACT SP/SR program, you will have the opportunity to consider where to focus your efforts. You may choose to work with areas of personal or professional life and concentrate on your freely chosen values in either area. Of course, it is possible to focus on more than one problem, domain of life, or valued aim during this work. However, it is important that you monitor yourself and choose aims that are appropriate to the time you have, the context of your SP/SR work, and your personal capacity.

In general, it is suggested, if you are new to ACT or therapy in general, that you focus your SP/SR aims on work-related values, such as your development as an ACT therapist, the challenges of being a trainee or student, or conflicting demands in your training context. If you are experienced with ACT, you may find more nuanced or personal aims more beneficial. This could include personal valued aims from work or other areas of living. Work aims might include working with clients with complex presenting problems, challenging experiences of countertransference arising in supervision, or conflicting demands between work and other valued domains.

Time Management and Planning

Given that this workbook's exercises sequentially build on one another, the modules of the ACT SP/SR program are recommended to be completed in sequential order. Prior to beginning your SP/SR program it is important that you plan to spend a sufficient amount of time completing the exercises and engaging in reflection. This means planning the amount of calendar time over which you will be working on ACT SP/SR. For example, a group might choose to work together for a period of 12–14 weeks, planning times and dates for their meetings in advance, as well as discussing their own, individual time management plans for completion of portions of the workbook. It may also be helpful to schedule regular, specific times for solitary work to complete the workbook modules and to compose written reflections. Planning for this time at regularly scheduled periods, without leaving long gaps of time between modules, can help with effective learning, focusing, and maintaining motivation throughout the process.

It is suggested that each module should be completed, including reflections, over the course of a week, or 2 weeks in group SP/SR. Each module should take anywhere from 2 to 3 hours, depending on the content and the individual. Some of the exercises in the modules require frequent or daily practices. Others involve longer periods of reflection. In general, it is suggested that the program take no less than 16–18 weeks to complete. Planning ahead with a realistic expectation for time commitments will increase the likelihood for your successful completion of your ACT SP/SR program.

Choosing When to Do SP/SR

Given the time commitment and self-focused nature of the ACT SP/SR program, it is suggested to not begin your program during a highly stressful or challenging period of your life. ACT SP/SR is about *learning* ACT from the inside out, and this is not really "self-therapy." This kind of learning may be more effective when an individual is not under conditions of significant threat or distress, and if significant stress or disturbances are present, it may be best to wait to begin your SP/SR work at another time. If this is not possible, for instance, if SP/SR is a program requirement, then choosing aims that are only mildly challenging is recommended. However, we often do not choose when stress and challenges might arrive in our lives. In fact, we have had to address some very significant and unplanned challenges while we were working through our own ACT SP/SR programs. We wound up facing personal losses, medical problems, and extremely stressful circumstances, all unexpected, right in the middle of our neatly planned ACT SP/SR journey. In addition to our own personal support systems, supervision, and psychotherapy, we found that the supportive context of an ACT SP/SR group, coupled with the powerful transformational potential of ACT techniques, were helpful resources as we worked through some of the more difficult stressors that we have known. After all, we are all in the same boat, and we all face the ubiquity of human suffering together. It is one thing to know how to build a fire, to have that knowledge in the mind, and to still shiver in the cold night with dry logs and an empty fireplace. It is quite another to actually build that fire and to tend to its warmth and light when we need it. SP/SR methods can bring us back to the evidence-based tools that we have learned in a more structured and personal way, inviting us to direct our expertise and compassion inward, supporting the therapists themselves, as they continue to share their strength with others.

Encouraging Confidentiality

If you are participating in ACT SP/SR in some form of group format, it is important for you to remember that "how" and "what" you choose to share with others is *your choice and you are in control of what and when you share*. Sometimes we can benefit from planning intentional pauses and "moments of mindfulness" when we might give ourselves the time and space to make choices about what we discuss and disclose. Using these moments to slow down and act with purpose and deliberate intention is particularly relevant when we are caught up in an emotionally charged flow of action and group process. In ACT SP/SR, we generally recommend making a distinction between the content of personal reflections, which might be written for you alone, and public or group shared reflections. Your private reflections are for your eyes only, and can go into the depth of your experience, thoughts, and feelings (reflective processes are covered in the "Building Your Reflective Capacity" section in this chapter). The material in the reflections that you share in any context, however, is up to you. It is generally suggested that your shared reflection be focused on the process of your experience rather than the in-depth content of your personal reflections.

Developing a Personal Support Strategy

The nature and processes involved in ACT SP/SR commonly raise some challenging or tough experiences for the participants. Learning ACT from the inside out can involve facing challenges, and this often involves feeling discomfort and facing things that are difficult. This is a part of the process. However, there may be times when something may be more challenging or personally triggering for you, and it is important that you have effective access to any help or support you require. This is why it is recommended that everyone complete a personalized, graded series of steps and resources for support in the event of significant distress or difficulty prior to beginning the program.

Here is a typical example of a Personal Support Strategy:

- Seek support and discuss the difficulty with a partner, psychotherapist, competent confidante from your support network, or trusted ACT SP/SR colleague. It is good to identify these people as support resources in advance of beginning your ACT SP/SR work, and to have their consent and commitment to help should the need arise before you begin the work.
- Speak with the SP/SR facilitator about the difficulty that is arising.
- If difficulties persist longer than 2–3 weeks, and you are not already working with a psychotherapist, it is suggested that you meet with a qualified, licensed, and identified local psychotherapist or mental health professional for further support.

Summary: Practicalities of ACT SP/SR— Maximizing Engagement and Reaping the Benefits

- Choose appropriate aims for ACT SP/SR based on time, context, and capacity. This typically includes identifying a problem to work with for SP/SR focus.
- Choose the focus of SP/SR aims: professional or personal.
- Work with intense personal trauma and deeply challenging clinical problems solely through SP/SR is not recommended (Bennett-Levy et al., 2015). Exercise self-care and seek professional help if you are dealing with active substance misuse, intrusive trauma-related problems, psychotic symptoms, or a severe mood disorder and are engaging in ACT SP/SR.
- Plan time, space, and schedule for ACT SP/SR meetings and individual work.

- Choose effective timing to begin, knowing that it isn't optimal to begin this work during times of intense personal distress or crisis.
- Establish confidentiality agreements and distinguish what to include in personal versus shared reflections.
- Prior to beginning your ACT SP/SR program, develop a Personal Support Strategy.

Building Your Reflective Capacity

The process of SR can be a powerful experience. The act of reflection we are referring to involves observing and understanding our experiences in ACT SP. There is significant variability in individual differences in the capacity and motivation for SR (Sanders & Bennett-Levy, 2010). Some individuals are innately motivated and skilled in SR, while others may not be as motivated or have not had the opportunities to develop these skills. There are many factors that can influence this capacity, such as conflicting demands from other valued domains of living. The pressures of busily "living life on life's terms" can reduce the likelihood that we engage in effective and consistent SR—this process is key in ACT SP/SR. Therefore, we provide some guidelines for cultivating and engaging in SR. This includes preparation for the reflection process, engaging in SR, reflection writing, and how to care for yourself through the process.

Preparing for Reflection

The following guidelines and tips are for establishing a safe, manageable, and sustainable structure that facilitates an effective reflection process:

- Schedule and commit to a regular time for reflection. As mentioned in the section on time management, setting and committing to a time frame for SP/SR helps ensure continued motivation and successful completion.

- Be aware that strong emotional responses may arise. SP/SR can elicit a range of emotions. At times, it can be uncomfortable or distressing, and at others, exciting, exhilarating, or joyful. The designers of SP/SR emphasize that there is no right or wrong way to experience your process (Bennet-Levy et al., 2015). Everyone has different responses and responds differently at different times and to different modules.

- Prepare for blocks. Blocks, resistance, or urges to avoid can be expected in ACT SP/SR. Examples of these include experiences of ambivalence or urges to give up entirely. When these show up, see whether you can use the practices and exercises in the modules to focus on the experience of feeling blocked. It is suggested that you plan ahead for how you might effectively respond to possible blocks. For example, practicing defusion from the thoughts surrounding these blocks and making a value-based choice as to what to do next can help. This in itself is an example of using ACT methods as a part of your own SP. In this way, every block or element of "resistance" can be a part of the process of self-development to which you have committed. You can also seek support and guidance from those in your personal support plan or other members of your SP/SR group.

• Prepare for possible breaks in the process. As best you can, take care to minimize distractions and disruptions to the SP/SR process and program. Life happens, and interruptions such as vacations, illness, or other unexpected events will arise. However, if we respond and plan flexibly, we can often continue to honor our commitments even in the presence of practical obstacles. If breaks are unavoidable, taking steps to ensure reengagement, commitment, and continuity are essential. If this is done in a group context, clarity of expectations, definitive communication, and shared commitment about beginning again will be helpful. When working on our own, clearly specifying the parameters of our commitments to ourselves can be very useful.

• Keep your workbook and reflection materials in a safe and accessible place. Choose a place to keep your SP/SR workbook and reflections where they are easy to get to and for you to feel secure in terms of confidentiality.

Engaging in the Process of Reflection

When it is time for written reflections, consider the following recommendations:

• Find a time and space with minimal distraction and disruptions. Identify a place to engage in the SR process that feels comfortable and free from distractions. Do your best to minimize the likelihood that your work will be disturbed.

• Use a centering or transitional practice. Prior to engaging in the SR or when transitioning from SP to SR, it is suggested you engage in a centering exercise, focused breathing, or mindfulness practice.

EXERCISE. Centering

This centering exercise can be practiced prior to engaging with the SR questions. An audio copy of this exercise may be downloaded from the book's website (see the box at the end of the table of contents).

As you begin, allow your eyes to close. Now, gently direct your attention to the sounds around you in the room. If it is quiet, or even silent, just notice the absence of sound, sensing the space around you. When you are ready, bring your attention to the sounds outside of the room. Next, direct your attention to the sounds even farther away than that. On your next natural inhalation, draw your attention to the physical sensations you experience here and now, sitting in this relaxed posture. See whether you can allow your attention to settle on your breath. As you breathe in, observing whatever sensations emerge in your awareness. As you exhale, simply let go of that awareness as the breath leaves the body. With each breath, noticing whatever sensations are present. Allowing the breath to find its own pace and breathe itself. Allowing awareness of any changes in sensation as the cycle of breathing continues. As you do this, remain aware that there is no need to change this experience in any way. If you notice your mind wandering, remember that is the nature of what minds do. Gently return your attention to the flow of your breathing. From time to time, it may be helpful to ground yourself in the present moment by feeling the physical sensations that you are experiencing. In doing this, you may connect with the sensations of the feet or knees on the ground, your seat on your chair or cushion, your spine, which is straight and supported, and the flow of the breath in and out of the body. Continue this practice in this manner for a few moments. Before letting go of this practice, you may again bring your mindful attention to the sounds around you in the room, the sounds that are just outside the room, and the sounds that are farther away even than that. With your next natural inhale, when you are ready, open your eyes and begin your SR practice.

- Utilize strategies that help you enhance recall of your experiences and increase awareness of your private experiences, such as your thoughts and feelings. Some suggested strategies to help recall of events and experiences for ACT SP/SR reflection include:

    ○ **Closing your eyes.** When recalling an experience and tuning in to your private events and responses, closing your eyes in this moment can be useful.

    ○ **Using imagery.** When recalling a particular experience or event, see whether you can reconstruct the scene in your mind, using as much detail as possible, focusing on the details of the sensory experiences available. Examples include those things you could see such as what others were wearing and their facial expressions, and those things you could hear, such as their tone of voice, your tone of voice, other sounds around you, and elements of the environment or atmosphere.

    ○ **Tuning in to how you recall feeling, physically and emotionally.** Take the time to remember what was happening there and then during the practice, and what was going through your mind in the situation being recalled, as well as how you are feeling now in the process of recall.

    ○ **Taking opportunities for mindfulness and acceptance.** Spend time being with your thought and feelings. Take an opportunity to be with this experience, just as it is without rushing into problem solving or a "doing" mode. Remember that this is a time for reflection and not necessarily for action.

    ○ **Utilizing your observer self, maintaining curiosity, and noticing the unexpected.** SR is intended to be approached with an open and flexible perspective. Bring bare attention and nonjudgmental awareness to whatever arises during this process of reflection.

    ○ **Monitoring for psychological inflexibility**, such as *fusion* and *avoidance* processes. Take notice of how you are reflecting, or if you are reexperiencing, ruminating, worrying, or criticizing instead.

    ○ **Practicing self-compassion and being your own compassionate facilitator.** If you notice yourself being overly critical or judgmental with yourself, use this as an opportunity to practice self-compassion. ACT SP/SR can involve noticing our struggle—responding to this struggle with wisdom and commitment is what learning ACT from the inside out is about.

○ **Remembering that SR is a process and can come in waves.** There may be times when you feel stuck or obstacles arise that prevent the SR process. You can always put the reflections aside and come back at a later time, when inspiration strikes or when you feel ready to give it another go.

○ **Looking for opportunities for generalizing valued learning and insights.** ACT SP/SR aims to help participants discover linkages between the professional and the personal domains of their lives. Research on SP/SR suggests that participants who reported the most benefit from the program reflected on themselves in both professional and personal contexts (Bennett-Levy & Lee, 2014).

○ **Using the reflection questions to guide you.** At the end of each module there are SR questions. They are there to help guide your written reflections. We suggest that you ask yourself these questions and feel free to add your own. The intention is to help enrich and deepen your understanding and help you make connections, relating your insights to your experience of yourself, your clients, and your work in ACT or other valued areas of living.

SR Writing

• Write in the first person. ACT SP/SR is personal and self-focused, as are the written reflections. Thus, it is suggested to write in the first person and from your perspective. The intention here is to not distance yourself from your experience but to get inside, observe, and reflect on it.

• Your writing is for you, not an audience. Try not to edit yourself—write openly and honestly.

• Writing provides an opportunity for perspective taking and new insights. In ACT SP/SR, written SR "writing is not the product of thinking; writing *is* thinking" (Bennett-Levy et al., 2015, p. 23). Through this process, participants discover new ways of perceiving their experience and often reach new insights and understandings.

Taking Care of Yourself

• Keep yourself and your individual aims in mind and take care of your needs. You are the expert on you and what you need in a given moment. Take good care of yourself through this process, using your time and energy with ACT SP/SR in a manner that meets your needs and is in service of your personal aims.

• Remember, there is no right or perfect way to do this.

CHAPTER 4

Guidance for Facilitators

Making the commitment to facilitate an ACT SP/SR group has many benefits and important responsibilities. Sharing a process of knowledge discovery and enabling colleagues as they access new perspectives can be very rewarding and meaningful. The process of facilitating an ACT SP/SR group can also provide deeper understanding and personal learning on the part of the facilitator. While these benefits and experiences are similar to those of other forms of group leading or teaching, as we will see, there are some differences and distinctions that make being an ACT SP/SR facilitator a unique and noteworthy experience. The purpose of this chapter is to provide guidance for those of you who intend to serve as ACT SP/SR group facilitators. However, even if you do not intend on being a group facilitator, you may still find this chapter a significant, but not an essential, component for your ACT SP/SR program. This chapter will help the facilitator adapt the groups to maximize the benefit for everyone involved.

ACT SP/SR groups can vary in context and size. Some examples of possible ACT SP/SR groups are peer-led groups, trainer-led groups in professional development settings, or groups established in other existing ACT-based training programs. In this chapter, we review the facilitator's responsibilities and provide a guide to tailor your group to effectively work in a way that is feasible for your specific context and meets the participants' individual aims. This chapter is divided into four sections, which relate to (1) the role and tasks of the ACT SP/SR facilitator, (2) aligning the ACT SP/SR program with participants' experiences and needs, (3) preparation for ACT SP/SR, and (4) maintaining group motivation and maximizing benefit for each of the participants.

The Role of the ACT SP/SR Facilitator

Those of us who have attended an ACT workshop or training can attest to how personal, experiential, and often powerful these learning experiences can be. So, there is no surprise that the experience of facilitating an ACT SP/SR group offers something similar and can take these meaningful learning experiences further. Through SP/SR, we get inside and inhabit the processes of ACT. We remain open to applying this ACT-consistent focus to any or all possible realms of living. The choice of where to apply this focus lies with each participant. The ACT SP/SR model is open and flexible, not overly rigid or limited by particular teaching points or curriculum. Ultimately, it is the facilitator who creates the conditions and provides guidance for the work to unfold and flourish.

In the context of SP/SR, we use the descriptive title of "facilitator" rather than trainer, group leader, or therapist. The role of an ACT SP/SR facilitator is similar to that of an ACT trainer or group leader, with some significant differences. Facilitating an ACT SP/SR program or group necessitates both similar and different skill sets to that of training ACT or leading an ACT group (Bennett-Levy et al., 2015). Both the traditional views of ACT training and ACT SP/SR are flexible, grounded in CBS, and involve a large component of experiential learning. Typically, in ACT trainings, the focus is on the development of the individuals' clinical capacities or an increase in their abilities to "do ACT." In contrast, in ACT SP/SR there is a stronger focus on the participants' unique personal struggles, with a wider array of choice as to what to focus their SP/SR work on and how to apply what they are learning in their lives. Additionally, in ACT SP/SR there is an ongoing group discussion forum between meetings, and written reflections are highly emphasized and encouraged by the facilitator.

The learning that transpires in ACT SP/SR is personal, experiential, and reflective by nature. This requires a safe context and an effective group process. There are several central ways in which the ACT SP/SR facilitator cultivates this type of context with the group—it begins with the facilitator's awareness of the needs of each participant. As always, collaborative relationships are key and the SP/SR facilitator maintains an open and collaborative relationship with the group and its members. The facilitator fosters support and safeness by helping participants understand the rationale, process, and commitments involved in the SP/SR group and ensures their informed consent and individual commitments.

The facilitator creates the conditions that increase effective group cohesion, interaction, and learning. This includes certain structures of the group, such as the scheduling, communication, and collaboration processes. ACT SP/SR groups are intended to go on for several weeks to months to provide the time and continuity for this context and work to progress and practice to deepen with reflection. The facilitator is responsible for communicating the schedule to the groups and providing any additional information or support necessary for ongoing group functioning.

Facilitators also function as an observer for the group and its process. They mindfully observe and monitor for blocks to the group and individual participants' interpersonal process, progress, and intrapersonal change process. ACT SP/SR group facilitators are engaged, open, and aware in the group process. They set up a context for discussion, actively observing and providing feedback. They monitor for both processes of psychological flexibility and inflexibility in the group and its participants. For example, the facilitator utilizes opportunities for pause when the group or one of its members is engaging in behaviors that interfere with established aims or group values. Alternatively, if there is noticeable change or a significant embodiment of values and meeting of aims, the facilitator will take an opportunity to highlight this. The role of the facilitator as an observer is to notice and highlight group and individual obstacles or blocks and progress, such as the positive movement in valued directions or successful approximations of individual aims. Essentially, the facilitator serves as a conscious social reinforcer, choosing responses mindfully that will shape more adaptive and values-directed behaviors among the group.

The following sections provide the details and expand on the key factors involved in the facilitator's responsibilities and give suggestions for successfully creating a safe context for your ACT SP/SR group.

Summary: The Roles and Responsibilities of the ACT SP/SR Facilitator

- Establishing and maintaining a safe context.
  - Cultivating collaborative relationships with participants.
- Helping participants understand the rationale and process involved.
  - Ensuring participants' informed consent and individual commitments.
- Fostering an effective group process.
  - Creating structure, scheduling, and communication.
  - Serving as a social reinforcer of adaptive and values-consistent behaviors.
- Functioning as an observer for the group and its process.
  - Monitoring for psychological flexible and inflexible processes.

Aligning the ACT SP/SR Program with Participants' Competencies and Needs

ACT SP/SR groups and processes aim to embody psychological flexibility and can be easily modified or adjusted to meet the demands of effective group processes and the specific needs of each group member. These adjustments can be made by adapting or refocusing certain aspects of the program or even by adding additional material when needed. The factors to consider when adapting an ACT SP/SR program to meet participants' needs include both environmental and personal factors. Some of these to consider are the context in which the program is taking place, the participant's knowledge of ACT, the scope of the ACT SP/SR program's focus (such as a focus on the "therapist self," "personal self," or "multiple selves"), and the individual's capacity to engage in SR processes.

ACT SP/SR groups can take many different forms and its members will have varying levels of experience and, of course, unique personal histories. As a facilitator, it is your role to work through a program that is in line with the needs and competencies of the group members with whom you are working. You won't need to reinvent the wheel and stray too far from the material in this workbook. However, it is a good idea to intentionally tailor the approach and even the intellectual or emotional tone of your group meetings to the style and expertise level of your group. In general, SP/SR groups aim to be flexible and able to adapt appropriately to different contexts.

Of course, some groups function in the context of an introductory-level ACT training, while others take place in more advanced training or peer consultation settings. In service of group coherence, it is a general SP/SR principle that groups be homogeneous in terms of clinical skills and relevant competencies experience when possible (Bennett-Levy et al., 2001). Examples of clinical skills and relevant competencies for ACT SP/SR facilitators to consider for group coherence include knowledge of ACT theory and practice, clinical experience, understanding and fluency with RFT concepts, and the participants' reflective capacities and skills.

Clearly, the stage of development of the therapist in terms of knowledge of ACT theory and practice and clinical experience will inform how the facilitator focuses the SP/SR program. For individuals early in their clinical career or brand new to ACT, there will be a focus on helping establish and transfer declarative or factual knowledge of ACT and its theory to procedural or experiential knowledge, putting ACT into action. When we grow and learn through an intellectual, artistic, or spiritual discipline, we begin with innocence, proceed through knowledge acquisition, cultivate ourselves through practice, and move toward mastery of internalized procedures. Mastery has been said to represent the presence of innocence in the context of experience. In this way, part of the facilitator's challenge and charge rests in creating contexts that allow for present-moment-focused spontaneity, while affording opportunities for repetition leading to masterful execution of technique. The core processes of ACT are experiential in nature and so this form of procedural learning is key at any level of training (Hayes et al., 2012). However, for clinicians who are newer to clinical work and ACT, facilitators may want to focus this work on their "therapist self." For participants who are more experienced with ACT, the scope of the SP/SR program can be wider, to include other aspects of themselves and their lives. For instance, in other SP/SR programs, more seasoned clinicians have focused their program on enhancing and expanding self-awareness, interpersonal skills, and increasing reflective capacity (Davis, Thwaites, Freeston, & Bennett-Levy, 2015).

The series of questions you will find at the end of each forthcoming module serve as a guide for the written SR component of this program. Facilitators can easily tailor the workbook's curriculum to the needs of a given group or individual by simply changing these questions to match the particular focus or scope of their work. Learning ACT from the inside out is all about enabling participants to embody their values and become more of who they want to be. Accordingly, facilitators can feel free to adjust these materials in ways that suit their focus, without altering the core processes involved or the structure of the program.

Another way of matching the ACT SP/SR program to participants' competencies and needs is by providing additional or supplemental training and support. This could be in the form of declarative and theoretical knowledge for those newer in learning ACT. Other supplemental learning might include those peer-reviewed articles and texts that relate to a particular interest or focus of the ACT SP/SR group. For example, if the ACT SP/SR program was focused for those individuals working with a particular population or aspect of human suffering, supplemental materials might include information on pertinent or related ACT approaches. Many resources can be found by searching the area of interest on the home page of ACBS (*www.contextualscience.org*).

Facilitators might also choose to invite participants to deepen their experiential practice through adding guided meditations, imagery practices, and ACT techniques not specified in this program. While each of the modules for the ACT SP/SR program have experiential practices directed at a particular ACT process, ACT is far more than a toolbox approach. The focus of ACT SP/SR should be on the underlying processes of psychological flexibility rather than the mastery of a range of tools, tips, or tricks. Any of the illustrative techniques in this workbook are meant to bring the participants into close contact with these core processes. Eventually, skilled ACT therapists will be able to deploy a range of different techniques to shape the processes of psychological flexibility and will even be able to improvise new techniques suited to the needs of given clients. As a result, ACT SP/SR facilitators and participants need not be limited to the techniques included in the modules.

As we have seen, the participants' individual needs, their level of knowledge and experience with ACT, and the context of the SP/SR group itself all inform how the facilitator can help align the needs of the participants with the appropriate scope and adaptations of the ACT SP/SR work. The facilitator, taking into consideration the context and needs of the group and its members, can adjust the program to have a wide or narrow focus and match the program with the participants' experience and valued aims for their work.

Summary: Aligning the ACT SP/SR Program with Participants' Competencies and Needs— Considerations for Adapting the SP/SR Program

- The context in which the program is taking place.
- The participants' knowledge and experience of ACT.
- Determining the scope of the SP/SR program's focus ("therapist self," "personal self," or multiple selves/"hybrid").
- Providing supplemental training or support (for theoretical, context/focus-specific, experiential, or reflective learning).

Preparation for ACT SP/SR

The preparation process is an important element to ensuring a successful ACT SP/SR program. The facilitator is responsible for navigating this process and guiding participants through the program. There are two key components or strategies to this preparatory process: (1) preparing a program prospectus and (2) holding a preprogram meeting (Bennett-Levy et al., 2015). The creators of the SP/SR approach note that a preparatory process with these two strategies in use increase the likelihood for participants' motivation and engagement (Bennett-Levy et al., 2015).

Program Prospectus and Preprogram Meeting

A program prospectus and preprogram meeting are intended to provide informed consent, enhance commitment, and increase the engagement of the participants. While the needs of each group will result in a different prospectus and meeting, there are a few things that are essential components in the preprogram process. Similar to the discussion of informed consent for clients in therapy, it is important to provide participants in ACT SP/SR with a clear understanding of what it is they are making a commitment to, answer any questions they might have, and correct any misgivings or misunderstandings about what to expect. As we mentioned earlier, this is part of creating a safe environment. The program prospectus and preprogram meeting are also intended to provide the participants with clear and useful information regarding the nature of ACT SP/SR work.

The program prospectus is designed to address questions about ACT SP/SR in advance. Such questions will naturally involve elements like safety, confidentiality, and empirical support for SP/SR programs. The prospectus should be distributed to program participants prior to the preprogram meeting, ideally giving the participants a few weeks to review it. For example, a participant who is completely new to SP/SR work may have questions as basic as "Why should someone consider an ACT SP/SR program and what can be expected?" Providing a clear and motivating rationale for the choice to join an ACT SP/SR program is indeed important for clarity of consent and motivation to engage. The prospectus' rationale for ACT SP/SR should be drawn from a blend of up-to-date research findings on ACT and on SP/SR in general, leading trainers' and clinicians' advocacy for experientially based learning, and examples of prior participants' reflections and testimony. These elements can be reflected in an original prospectus created by the facilitator, summarizing some of the material in this book with recent advances in the literature that will emerge over time. Alternatively, the facilitator may simply choose to suggest that participants read Chapters 1–3 of this workbook, perhaps adding some reflections shared by prior participants of other ACT SP/SR programs, if available.

The preprogram meeting provides an in-person opportunity for the facilitator to elaborate on the information in the prospectus, bridging didactic knowledge with practice. This meeting provides an opportunity for the group to share questions, review, and make adjustments to the program to fit the participants' needs. The facilitator's role in this meeting is to be as open and flexible in tailoring the SP/SR program to fit the context and individual participants as possible. For instance, the meeting can provide more information regarding the previous experiences of prior participants and what it's like to experience ACT from the inside out. Some facilitators have even asked prior participants to drop in on a new preprogram meeting to answer questions and share aspects of their experience with SP/SR. The facilitator may also discuss the role of SP/SR in learning and ongoing cultivation of particular ACT skills and processes, the effectiveness and importance of experiential and reflective learning in SP/SR, and the capacity and integrative nature of SP/SR programs.

Creating Clear and Agreed-Upon Program Requirements

The SP/SR program requirements will vary depending on context and participants' collaborative agreements—thus, as we have suggested, the facilitator should be as flexible and open as possible in order to accommodate these needs and differences in restrictions. The facilitator provides a clear and informed understanding of the core structure of the SP/SR program and collaboratively with the group creates the agreements. The preprogram meeting needs to allow enough time to come to a collaborative agreement regarding the following: expectations regarding commitments, contributions, confidentiality, and safety (the latter two are discussed in the next section).

In terms of commitment and contribution of participants, the group should reach an agreement regarding the requirements for written reflections. Are they to be completed after every module? What are the deadlines for posting reflections? Are participants required to take part in a discussion forum? What form or structure is involved in the reflection process? What happens when a participant is unable to complete the reflections?

The next topic for discussion is how much time is required in an SP/SR program. How much time does each participant need to successfully complete modules? Facilitators need to help the group schedule a sufficient amount of time for participants to realistically engage in SP/SR and group-related discussions involved in an ACT SP/SR program. The creators of this approach suggest a minimum of 2–3 hours per module of individual time for the participant and, depending on the requirements of the module, 1–3 weeks to complete a module as a group (Bennett-Levy et al., 2015). Facilitators are asked to consider and suggest appropriate timing and a schedule for the implementation of each module.

SP/SR programs have previously been implemented over the course of 12–24 weeks or one or two semesters in a university or graduate setting (Bennett-Levy & Lee, 2014; Bennett-Levy et al., 2015). If your SP/SR program is a part of a larger clinical training program, then it is recommended that you align your schedule and structure with the core curriculum. The form of experiential and reflective learning involved in ACT SP/

SR is maximized when this practice occurs shortly after trainees are exposed to the didactic or declarative information on a particular technique or skill through readings, lectures, or workshops. Thus, matching content with a larger training curriculum helps provide effective structure and progression of an SP/SR program.

Finally, in terms of commitment and contribution, the groups must discuss whether assessments of any form will be used or whether they are required by the context in which the SP/SR program is being offered. Currently, there are no evidence-based approaches for the assessment of SP/SR—its creators suggest the use of outcome measures associated with particular SP/SR program learning objectives and targets. Context-specific or institutional requirements may also impact how attendance will be handled. The groups should collaboratively agree upon attendance expectations and exceptions, to the extent that this is possible. Facilitators should ensure that the group is aware of any assessment, attendance, or other institutional or context-specific requirements.

Creating a Feeling of Safety with the Process

The third essential component of the program prospectus and preprogram meeting is creating a sense of safety with the ACT SP/SR program. As we mentioned in the previous section, this involves issues of confidentiality and security. The program prospectus should provide a clear overview of the process of SP/SR and of the preprogram meeting. During the meeting, it is important for the facilitator to elicit participants' concerns and fears. For example, the facilitator can ask about participants' concerns about the program or their involvement. After making room for everyone to voice their concerns, the facilitator can invite the group to offer suggestions as to how to address these concerns. If it does not arise, the facilitator can bring up issues of confidentiality and anonymity. The group members should discuss how they would like to handle issues of anonymity and confidentiality. Again, remembering to remain open and flexible to the needs and context of the group, the facilitator helps the group reach an agreement on how rigid or flexible these boundaries are. Some examples of questions to address here include "Will the shared reflections be anonymous or do participants want to use their real names?" and "What can be discussed outside of group?" These agreements should be documented and made available to all involved.

The facilitator uses the opportunity of the prospectus and the preprogram meeting to emphasize and discuss the distinctions in form and function between material in private reflections and public reflections. When it comes to public reflections—those written reflections that participants share in the forum and group discussions—participants are instructed to focus on functional or process content and their experiences or observations of the process being explored, not necessarily the personal content of the material. An example of a public "function-focused" reflection is "I noticed how much more difficult it was to practice defusion from my judgments than I expected it would be. I found myself feeling frustrated and critical of myself." Private ACT SP/SR reflections can include more personal content in the form of experiences or observations. For example, a private form-focused reflection follows: "Physically, I noticed tension and heat rising in my body, and my mind was telling me 'I am a phony.' These are typical experiences when I think that I will never be as good as my peers and that I should never be anyone's therapist. I felt like quitting and didn't talk much."

These distinctions provide the participants with some guidance and provides an opportunity for choosing how much and where to share their private experiences in written reflections.

The nature of the work involved in ACT SP/SR commonly raises some challenging or tough experiences for the participants. Thus, it would make sense that many participants have fears or concerns of what will happen when they come in contact with this. For some this may be fear of "losing control" or not having enough support. The facilitator might say something like the following to open up the discussion:

ACT from the inside out involves facing our challenges and expanding our abilities to move toward our valued aims. This often involves feeling discomfort and facing things that are difficult. This is a part of the growth process. However, there may be times when something may be more challenging or personally triggering for you. So, in the rare case that you are experiencing significant distress or difficulty, it is important that you have effective access to any help or support you require. This is why we have each individual complete a "Personal Support Strategy," a personalized, graded series of steps and resources for support in the event of significant distress or difficulty.

At the preprogram meeting it is recommended that the facilitator consider with the participants what their optimal area for focusing their individual ACT SP/SR program might be. For instance, the group might be invited to consider choosing their SP/SR focus in an area that is moderately challenging, but that they do not anticipate will be overwhelming, cause significant distress, or impede their practice and reflection.

Finally, facilitators address their own role in the group. Prior to the preparatory process, facilitators should consider what their intended role with the group will be by asking, "What are my roles and responsibilities in this group?"; "Will I participate in group or forum discussions?"; "If so, how?"; "Are there any dual relationships?"; and "If so, how will this be addressed?" Facilitators should then discuss these questions openly with the group, answer any questions that they may have, and together collaboratively form an agreement around the role and responsibilities of the facilitator.

Summary: ACT SP/SR Preparation

- The facilitator distributes the program prospectus and arranges a preprogram meeting.
- The program prospectus and preprogram meeting should include:
  - A specific, strong, and clear rationale for the SP/SR program.
  - Details of the ACT SP/SR program requirements and commitments.
  - Creating collaborative relationships and a supportive and safe group context.
- Confirm with group members that they develop a Personal Support Strategy.
- Clarify your role to the group and address any potential for dual relationships.

Creating an Enriching and Valuable Group Process

The ACT SP/SR program can be a meaningful and valued learning experience that often involves a connection to a learning community. The facilitator is responsible for cultivating and caring for SP/SR's enriching and supportive group process and cohesion. This community offers the opportunity for enriching dialogue, compassionate support, and moving interpersonal experiences. The SP/SR group discussion allows for multiple forms of perspective taking, expanding our understanding of ourselves, others, and the contexts in which we work and live. Groups also offer opportunities for social learning and modeling from the facilitator and other members. Learning ACT from the inside out with others allows for a cultivation of connection, community, and care for one another. As noted, even if you are completing this work without a typical SP/SR group, you are not alone, and others working through these modules, who are learning and living ACT, can be found on Facebook at *https://www.facebook.com/groups/actspsr*. The group may also seek to use its own social media or web-based resources for online meetings and blended learning. If you are an ACT SP/SR facilitator, then it is your job to help the group cultivate and maintain this supportive, enriching, and valuable group process throughout all of their in-person and online group communications.

The cultivation and care for group processes and helping participants get the most out of their ACT SP/SR group work continues through the duration of the program. Facilitators provide encouragement, support, and opportunities for answering participants' questions both in group meetings and between meetings. Ideally, facilitators are able to balance their role as an observer and provide feedback about the group process. Facilitators should be encouraging in their approach, supporting group participation, and helping the group continue to move toward shared values and aims.

Summary: Creating Enriching and Valuable Group Processes

- The group determines how and when to meet (i.e., online, face-to-face, or a combination).
- Facilitators determine their commitment to the group and together they collaboratively come up with expectations around group process and safety.
- The online discussion forum and meeting spaces should be easy to use and navigate.
- Facilitators encourage and support participation and help the group continue to move toward shared values and aims.

Looking After Individual Participants

In addition to caring for group processes and values, facilitators are also responsible for looking after individual participants and their unique process. As observers, facilitators commit to caring for the well-being of each of the participants. They monitor the participants and group discussions for individual struggle. Facilitators ensure that each participant has and uses their Personal Support Strategy when necessary. They also look out for participants' individual changes and successes. Again, balancing monitoring, observing, and providing feedback or guidance, facilitators are supportive and flexible in their approach.

As we have emphasized throughout this chapter, facilitators should be flexible and pragmatic in their approach, taking into account each participant—individual needs, aims, and above all, well-being. In order to do this, the facilitator establishes early on, perhaps in the preprogram meeting, how to best communicate and check in with each participant between group meetings. Together, the participant and facilitator can also decide whether and how this should be a part of the participant's Personal Support Strategy. The facilitator can also be flexible and make adjustments to the program for individual participants. For instance, when a group member is unable to participate fully at some point during the process, the facilitator might offer supplemental makeup material or changes in practice, attendance, or written reflection requirements. There may be times when continuing with the ACT SP/SR group may not be in a participant's best interest or may need to be changed in significant ways. The facilitator and participant can discuss what options are available for adaptations or whether taking a break or ending participation is appropriate. If struggle persists, the facilitator should contact the participant, discuss individual needs and the available options, and together decide on the next best steps. Ultimately, it is important to remember that consent and commitment to participate in an ACT SP/SR program, no matter the context, should be freely given by the participant and can be revoked or changed at any time. Participants should make an informed decision as to when it is best for them to begin the program. If ACT SP/SR is imbedded in a larger training program, university setting, or curricula, alternatives should be offered or adaptations made for individuals or situations where SP/SR participation is contraindicated.

Summary: Looking After Participants

- Monitor the participants and group discussions for individual struggle and successes.
- Facilitators ensure that each participant has a Personal Support Strategy.
- Facilitators are flexible, pragmatic, and individualized in their approach with each participant and their unique needs and values.
- SP/SR group participation and timing of the program should be a freely chosen informed decision made by participants or alternative pathways offered.

Concluding Comments

All of the preceding material provides the necessary background for you to organize, structure, and engage in an ACT SP/SR process as a group or as an individual. The following modules will be your roadmap through a gradual path of self-discovery based on ACT and CBS. We encourage you to engage with the following experientially and allow yourself the space and time to bring the power of your own insight and wisdom as a psychotherapist to working with yourself.

PART II

The ACT SP/SR Program

SECTION A

FACING THE CHALLENGE

Identifying and Formulating a Challenging Problem

It's now time for you to begin working through the modules of your SP/SR program. We are with you in our hearts and minds as well as in these words, and we can relate to what you must be experiencing. As we described earlier, we have worked through this ACT SP/SR approach, bringing this method to some great challenges in our lives. We also used ACT SP/SR to build new directions for ourselves and to enhance our own ability to pursue what matters most for us. Later in this chapter, we share some examples of our problem formulations, using the same forms and methods that you will use.

"We Begin Where We Are": My Baseline Measures

Similar to most systems of psychotherapy in the CBT family, measurement procedures are used in ACT. Thus, we suggest that you begin by establishing some baseline measurement procedures so that you can evaluate your progress. First, complete the Acceptance and Action Questionnaire–II (AAQ-II; Bond et al., 2011), a measure of psychological flexibility, the central hypothesized process of change in ACT (Hayes et al., 2012). Next, complete two general symptom severity measures: the Patient Health Questionnaire–9 (PHQ-9; Kroenke, Spitzer, & Williams, 2001) and the Generalized Anxiety Disorder seven-item scale (GAD-7; Spitzer, Kroenke, Williams, & Löwe, 2006). These are brief measures of emotional states, the former of depression and the latter of anxiety. While our ACT SP/SR program is not a form of psychotherapy, taking a new perspective of our current state of mind using psychometric tools is a good place to begin as we formulate our SP/SR work.

It's also very important that you keep in mind that *changing depression and/or anxiety scores on these (or other) scales is not the goal of ACT*. We point this out because our inclusion of these "symptom" measures might inadvertently smuggle the idea to you that direct change of mental experiences is our goal in ACT SP/SR.

It isn't.

So why have we included them?

Because these measures can provide you with useful information along your journey and your use of them replicates what clients experience in therapy. Our aim in ACT SP/SR is to cultivate psychological flexibility *in the service of living lives of meaning, purpose, and vitality.* Being aware of where our hearts and minds are at is helpful, and can provide a thread of awareness to help us along the road. Still, we aren't about getting inside your mind and culling out "bad" thoughts—rather, we are very much about *empowering you to take charge of your life,* and make it as beautiful, bold, and big as you wish.

After you've completed the AAQ-II, PHQ-9, and GAD-7, you'll identify a challenging problem to target during your SP/SR program. Finally, you'll construct an idiosyncratic measure that pertains to your challenging problem so that you can track your progress with respect to that problem across the program.

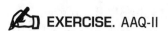 **EXERCISE.** AAQ-II

Pause for a moment now and complete, score, and interpret the AAQ-II using the instructions provided.

AAQ-II: PRE-SP/SR

Below you will find a list of statements. Rate how true each statement is for you by circling a number next to it. Use the scale below to make your choice.

1	2	3	4	5	6	7
never true	very seldom true	seldom true	sometimes true	frequently true	almost always true	always true

1. My painful experiences and memories make it difficult for me to live a life that I would value.	1 2 3 4 5 6 7
2. I'm afraid of my feelings.	1 2 3 4 5 6 7
3. I worry about not being able to control my worries and feelings.	1 2 3 4 5 6 7
4. My painful memories prevent me from having a fulfilling life.	1 2 3 4 5 6 7
5. Emotions cause problems in my life.	1 2 3 4 5 6 7
6. It seems like most people are handling their lives better than I am.	1 2 3 4 5 6 7
7. Worries get in the way of my success.	1 2 3 4 5 6 7

From Bond et al. (2011). Reprinted with permission from Frank W. Bond in *Experiencing ACT from the Inside Out: A Self-Practice/Self-Reflection Workbook for Therapists* by Dennis Tirch, Laura R. Silberstein-Tirch, R. Trent Codd, III, Martin J. Brock, and M. Joann Wright (The Guilford Press, 2019). Purchasers of this book can download additional copies of this form (see the box at the end of the table of contents).

This is a one-factor measure of psychological inflexibility, or experiential avoidance. Score the scale by summing the seven items. Higher scores equal greater levels of psychological inflexibility. The average (mean) score in a clinical population was 28.3 (*SD* 9.9), while in a nonclinical population it was 18.51 (*SD* 7.05). Scores of > 24–28 suggest probable current clinical distress and make future distress and functional impairment more likely (Bond et al., 2011).

✍️ EXERCISE. PHQ-9 and GAD-7

Next, complete the PHQ-9 and the GAD-7, and score and interpret them using the guidelines we provide below.

PHQ-9: PRE-SP/SR

Over the last 2 weeks, how often have you been bothered by the following problems?	Not at all	Several days	More than half the days	Nearly every day
1. Little interest or pleasure in doing things	0	1	2	3
2. Feeling down, depressed, or hopeless	0	1	2	3
3. Trouble falling or staying asleep, or sleeping too much	0	1	2	3
4. Feeling tired or having little energy	0	1	2	3
5. Poor appetite or overeating	0	1	2	3
6. Feeling bad about yourself—or that you are a failure or have let yourself or your family down	0	1	2	3
7. Trouble concentrating on things, such as reading the newspaper or watching television	0	1	2	3
8. Moving or speaking so slowly that other people could have noticed; or the opposite—being so fidgety or restless that you have been moving around a lot more than usual	0	1	2	3
9. Thoughts that you would be better off dead or of hurting yourself in some way	0	1	2	3

After completing the above measure, simply sum your score. The table on the next page explains how your score compares to how others with varying levels of depression and distress have scored.

0–4:	No indication of depression		
5–9:	Indicative of mild depression		
10–14:	Indicative of moderate depression		
15–19:	Indicative of moderately severe depression		
20–27:	Indicative of severe depression		
	My score: _____		

GAD-7: PRE-SP/SR

Over the last 2 weeks, how often have you been bothered by the following problems?	Not at all	Several days	More than half the days	Nearly every day
1. Feeling nervous, anxious, or on edge	0	1	2	3
2. Not being able to stop or control worrying	0	1	2	3
3. Worrying too much about different things	0	1	2	3
4. Trouble relaxing	0	1	2	3
5. Being so restless that it is hard to sit still	0	1	2	3
6. Becoming easily annoyed or irritable	0	1	2	3
7. Feeling afraid as if something awful might happen	0	1	2	3

Copyright by Pfizer, Inc. Reprinted in *Experiencing ACT from the Inside Out: A Self-Practice/Self-Reflection Workbook for Therapists* by Dennis Tirch, Laura R. Silberstein-Tirch, R. Trent Codd, III, Martin J. Brock, and M. Joann Wright (The Guilford Press, 2019). This form is free to duplicate and use. Purchasers of this book can download additional copies of this form (see the box at the end of the table of contents).

As you did with the previous measure, simply sum your score for the above items. The table below tells you how your score compares to others who have completed this same measure, with varying levels of anxiety present in their lives.

Scores of:			
0–4:	No indication of anxiety		
5–9:	Indicative of mild anxiety		
10–14:	Indicative of moderate anxiety		
15–21:	Indicative of severe anxiety		
	My score: _____		

After completing these measures, we suggest that you reflect on your scores and what they might mean for you. If you find that you are in a clinically relevant or severe range of depression, anxiety, or psychological inflexibility, we highly suggest that you discuss this with a trusted professional. You might choose to reach out to a supervisor, therapist, mentor, or colleague. If you are in therapy, share this information with your therapist. If you do not have mental health support, we suggest that you exercise self-compassion and seek the help that you need. This workbook and program is designed to help you deepen your psychotherapy practice and grow as a person. However, no workbook can be a substitute for the care and support that a qualified therapist, supervisor, or peer community can provide when facing difficult times.

If you have a specific concern not assessed by these severity measures (i.e., the PHQ-9 and the GAD-7), you should strongly consider exchanging them for other validated scales that directly assess your issues. For example, perhaps you are more concerned with anger, shame, lack of self-compassion, envy, and so on, rather than depression or anxiety. In this case, measurement tools specific to these issues will be of greater use to you. You can often find validated scales online that are in the public domain. Another source is the two-volume set *Measures for Clinical Practice and Research* (Corcoran & Fischer, 2013).

As you proceed through your ACT SP/SR program and complete each module, it would be useful for you to repeatedly use these assessment measures to track any observable changes in your degree of psychological flexibility, depression, and anxiety.

🖎 EXERCISE. "Where Do I Feel Stuck?": My Challenging Problem for the SP/SR Program

We therapists struggle with many of the same concerns as our clients, and our difficulties can emerge in both personal- and work-related contexts. In this exercise, you will identify a challenging problem to work on during the SP/SR program. One way of categorizing problems is into those that are about your "personal self" and those that are "professional self"—that is, those problems that primarily involve and influence your therapy work. SP/SR programs often separate problems into these two categories.

For our purposes as ACT practitioners, it's important that we hold these categories lightly. After all, a major part of psychological flexibility involves transcending attachment to your self-stories. There is a part of you that is more than, and different from, your narratives about your "personal self" and your "professional self." Still, this division can help us to focus in on a problem to address in our ACT SP/SR work. In this workbook, you may elect to identify a problem in either domain. We suggest that you think about which domain the problem you are choosing primarily involves, yet appreciate how interconnected all of the multiple domains of our lives can be.

For this exercise, it can be useful to find a quiet location and to begin with a brief period practicing mindful breathing. As you begin, allow yourself at least three mindful breaths, contacting the present moment and connecting with the experience of physical sensation in the body. In this moment, we are resting in the present and turning our attention inward, slowing the mind and slowing the body. Having gathered and centered your attention in this way, respond to the following steps.

1. Will the problem I choose involve primarily my "personal self" or my "professional self"?

2. If you selected a problem facing your "personal self," recall a time (the more recent, the better) when you were experiencing distress or ineffective behavior involving this problem. When you have accessed and experienced this memory, answer the following questions:

   • What was going on in this situation?

   • In what ways does this situation involve a recurring problem?

   • Does your life feel larger or smaller during such an experience? In what ways?

   • Does this difficulty sometimes intrude into your work with therapy clients?

   • If you were less involved in struggling with this problem, how would your life and therapy work be positively impacted?

3. If you just answered questions about a more personal problem, you can skip this step and proceed to Step 4. If you have decided to identify a problem primarily encountered in your work life, complete this step. Bring to mind a time when you encountered a particularly distressing experience and emotions in your work life. Perhaps you've noticed this experience with a certain clinical population or with a specific client. As you remember this experience, activate all of your senses. See what and who was there. Hear any sounds that were there. See whether you can feel what you were feeling there and then, here and now, in the body. Then ask yourself:

- What was going on in this situation?

- In what ways does this situation involve a recurring problem?

- Did my life feel larger or smaller during the experience? In what ways?

- Is this problem truly limited to my work life, or does it also show up in my personal life?

- If I were less involved in struggling with this problem, how would my life and therapy work be positively impacted?

4. The problem that I chose to work with through my ACT SP/SR program can be defined and described in the following way:

EXAMPLE: Dennis's Answers to "Personal" Problem Formulation Questions

- What was going on in this situation?
  When I have free time, often on the weekends, I feel like I would like to rest and relax after working a lot during the week. I sometimes choose to just chill out rather than continue with professional projects. This can trigger my feeling highly anxious and I can feel profound shame at such moments. My mind sometimes tells me stories about how I should be ashamed of myself for being behind in my tasks for work. I feel a relentless critic who tells me I'm not enough. This doesn't usually inspire me to take action, but rather discourages me. The time spent ruminating about why I am not working harder doesn't make me more productive, anyway. This just absorbs time that could be spent in relaxation, play, or work, and turns it into time spent focused on a struggle with my experience.

- In what ways does this situation involve a recurring problem?
  This is a problem that has been showing up in different contexts since I was 7 years old. It has to do with my trauma and abuse history beginning with childhood, at home and at school. I feel very driven to have meaningful experiences, and to accomplish things with the time I have on earth. When I feel I'm not living up to these aims, a cruel and discouraging inner critic can show up. My own personal therapy has pointed to a lot of causes and conditions in my learning history that have contributed to the problem too.

- Did my life feel larger or smaller during the experience? In what ways?
  My life feels much smaller. My past experiences feel devalued if I buy into this line of thinking. It's like I just can't access satisfaction and gladness in anything that I have accomplished in such moments. All of who I am is defined by a belief that I will never meaningfully progress with my responsibilities, and there is a lot of self-loathing. The joys of my current life don't seem as significant if I am absorbed by this shame-based perspective. The possibility of realizing my vision for the future feels diminished when this is my way of being.

- Is this problem truly limited to my work life, or does it also show up in my personal life?
  This particular problem doesn't show up in my work as a therapist in the consultation room, since it is triggered by my having freedom to choose my actions and relates to the possibility of just resting or of "doing nothing" for a little bit of time each week. While in a therapy session, I tend to have a more focused, mindful, and compassionate state of mind and body, and any of these kinds of thoughts, if they were even triggered, would be much less likely to "hook" me.

- If I were less involved in struggling with this problem, how would my life and therapy work be positively impacted?
  I really enjoy having some quiet time to rest and to relax, and sometimes such a period of unwinding or contemplation can provide space for deepening my experience and appreciation. I feel a yearning to feel safe and in a loving space with my family at home. If I were less hooked by this experience, I might be able to let go of the influence of stress and of my personal history of trauma and shame more fully, by engaging more deeply with the moment. What this means in practical terms is that I might have the freedom to take my life back and enjoy my time on earth more, with the people I love.

Self-Reflective Questions

Now that you have had the opportunity to take baseline measurements of your flexibility and some measures of your struggle, what have you noticed?

_____

_____

_____

_____

_____

_____

_____

_____

_____

_____

_____

_____

_____

Have you noticed any particular patterns that contribute to suffering and inflexibility in your life? If so, what might they be?

_____

_____

_____

_____

_____

_____

_____

_____

_____

_____

_____

_____

_____

How might your formulation of a problem area in your life relate to your work with your clients?

_____

_____

_____

_____

_____

_____

_____

_____

_____

_____

_____

_____

_____

_____

What have you learned in terms of your experience of yourself as a psychotherapist from this module?

_____

_____

_____

_____

_____

_____

_____

_____

_____

_____

_____

_____

MODULE 2

ACT SP/SR Challenge Formulation

Using the ACT SP/SR Challenge Formulation

Now that we have an initial definition of the problem you have chosen, we will refine your approach to the problem by looking more closely into the factors that contribute to this challenge. We approach the challenging situation you have chosen in several ways—in fact, our initial modules present a few different perspectives for the here and now. These include working with the ACT matrix and the hexaflex model of psychological flexibility. Our next step in formulating and approaching this problem involves our ACT SP/SR challenge formulation.

In some ways, the process of formulating a case may feel familiar to you. However, this time around, *you* are the "case" in question. Rather than turning outward and applying our method to some "other" at a distance, we are turning within and looking in a systematic way at how we are affected by a difficult experience. As we look deeper into the recurrent problem, you will likely find new ways of experiencing the challenge. For example, we will look at subtle dimensions of your relationship to the problem, including the intentions that may have been neglected in your life due to your absorption with this problem. As you proceed, as much as you can, bring the sensitivity and wisdom that you would bring to work with a valued client or friend to your work with yourself in ACT SP/SR.

The parts of this problem formulation consist of:

- The context.
- Your private experiences.
- How you are being "pulled by the future and/or pushed by the past."
- Valued intentions that are neglected/unrealized.
- Unhelpful avoidance and control behaviors.

The ACT SP/SR Challenge Formulation Summarized

In the practice that follows, we ask you to examine the problem you have chosen, and to describe it across five dimensions. Please review the previous exercise, and focus on the problem that you have identified and have begun to formulate. Think of a time when a strong emotional response to a situation related to this problem showed up. As much as you can, think about the situation in detail, including environmental factors, the immediate thoughts that arose, and thoughts that felt old and familiar. Consider how this experience might be connected to stories that you have told about your past self, or those you fear happening in the future. Also, consider what intentions you may have neglected as a result of responding to these stories, and what problematic behaviors resulted from this emotional experience.

The five factors we will think and write about include the following.

The Context

This is the situation in which the unwanted thoughts and emotional struggle occurred. This includes your physical location, who you were with, and the circumstance that triggered the thoughts, emotions, images, and sensations. As ACT has its roots in clinical behavioral analysis, we can understand the context as being the antecedent to subsequent overt and covert behavioral responses that may be a part of the problem.

My Private Experiences

These are the thoughts, images, or memories that unfold and proceed when we are in contact with this circumstance. This contact may be when we are directly in the context that triggers our responses, or this contact may be imaginal. For example, if I (Laura) historically have a pattern of fear and avoidance of public speaking, I may experience anticipatory anxiety and worry when I know that a speaking engagement is coming soon. I also may have direct fears and physical sensations related to threat perception that arise immediately before taking to the podium. These are the type of thoughts that "hook" us and exert a strong influence on our behavior and emotions when they arise. We essentially respond to these imaginal events as if they were real, and as if they were threatening to us in some sense. Accordingly, these thoughts affect our potential for psychological flexibility through our *fusion* with these thoughts. Furthermore, these are often thoughts that provoke experiential avoidance (EA) and unwillingness, leading to psychologically inflexible and constricted responses.

How I Am Being "Pulled by the Future and/or Pushed by the Past"

This factor represents the ways that our mental events cause us to lose contact with the present moment and the "here-and-now" contingencies that present themselves. When we are fused with worries about the future, obsessively problem solving potential "what-ifs" about our lives, we lose our connection to the presence. When we become immersed in ruminations and internal stimuli about our past regrets, or criticism of our actions, we are more involved with the imagined past than we are in responding to our present moment. Furthermore, in such moments, we are so absorbed by our personal narratives and our stories about who we are that we are typically far from the perspective of the "observing-self" frame of reference. In this way, the two central psychological flexibility processes involving *contact with the present moment* and *flexible perspective taking* are compromised when we are excessively pulled by the imagined future or pushed/dragged by the "remembered" past.

Valued Intentions That Are Neglected/Unrealized

We all have dreams and ambitions. We all wish to move toward lives of meaning and vitality. In ACT SP/SR, we recognize that certain qualities of doing and being are inherently reinforcing and become the valued intentions that bring purpose to our lives. We ask ourselves "What do I want to be about?"; "What do I want to stand for?"; and "What do I want to work toward in this life?"

Sometimes we work to realize our valued aims. At other times, avoidance or fusion with patterns of thinking can pull us away from showing up for our lives fully. For example, you may intend to be a reliable friend, but avoidance of feeling social anxiety pulls you away from gatherings, such as birthday parties or baby-naming ceremonies. You have lost the opportunity to share in your friend's happiness. You have also lost the opportunity to live as the version of yourself you most wish to be. In essence, your fusion and avoidance has turned you into a prisoner in your own life. Additionally, shame, guilt, and remorse about not being there for your friend can exacerbate the emotional pain in this struggle.

This factor asks you to look at what aims you are neglecting as a result of fusion with your thoughts about yourself or your life. What ways are you unable to keep commitments to yourself and others as you struggle with this problem area? This factor involves how clearly we can be the *authors of valued aims* in our lives, and how able and willing we are to *commit to action* in the realization of these values. These two components of psychological flexibility are central to the behavior change dimension of ACT.

Unhelpful Avoidance and Control Behaviors

At the heart of the ACT model of human suffering, we find our excessive efforts to avoid or overcontrol certain experiences. This factor represents an inventory of the behaviors we engage in that contribute to EA and the control agenda. These efforts typically backfire. We feel as though we can't stand to remember a recent breakup, so we may drink too much, and our ability to embody our values declines. We seek to avoid conflicts or rejections in our interpersonal relationships, so we isolate and have fewer rewarding experiences.

The philosophy of ACT is grounded on successful working as the determining factor in any analysis. As you complete this factor in the formulation, take some time to review the real-world behaviors you engage in around this problem.

- Where do you notice unhelpful or unworkable actions?
- Are there ways that you attempt to push away the problem, or suppress your emotions around this problem?
- Does this strategy lead to successful outcomes?
- How might you be engaging in unhelpful actions related to avoidance or overcontrol of your experiencing the problem?

Below, we provide a worksheet for you to complete an ACT SP/SR five-part formulation of the problem that you have chosen for this workbook. We begin with an example of how one of us (Joann) completed just such a formulation. Joann shares a five-part formulation that she used on her ACT SP/SR journey, in dealing with a recurrence of breast cancer.

 EXAMPLE: Joann's ACT SP/SR Challenge Formulation

The context
Finding out I had a breast cancer diagnosis, again.

My private experiences
I can't believe I have to go through this again.
I haven't been taking good enough care of my body.
I am so ashamed.
I drink alcohol and I know it increases the risk of breast cancer.
I should have worked out more often.
It's my fault.
I did this to myself.
I have let down my loved ones.

How I am being "pulled by the future and/or pushed by the past"
I wouldn't have cancer right now if I took better care of myself.
I did this to myself.
What if I continue this way?
More cancer?
If I talk about this with everyone, I will just bring them down, too.

Valued intentions that are neglected/unrealized
Being an available friend.
Self-care.
Being an engaged therapist.

Unhelpful avoidance and control behaviors
Assure friends and loved ones that "I am fine."
Increased alcohol consumption.
Decreased productivity.
Social isolation.

✍️ **EXERCISE.** My ACT SP/SR Challenge Formulation

```
┌──────────────────────────────────────────────────────────┐
│ The context                                               │
│                                                           │
│                                                           │
│                                                           │
│ My private experiences                                    │
│                                                           │
│                                                           │
│                                                           │
│ How I am being "pulled by the future and/or pushed by     │
│ the past"                                                 │
│                                                           │
│                                                           │
│                                                           │
│ Valued intentions that are neglected/unrealized           │
│                                                           │
│                                                           │
│                                                           │
│ Unhelpful avoidance and control behaviors                 │
│                                                           │
│                                                           │
└──────────────────────────────────────────────────────────┘
```

Developing a Problem Statement

Now that you have identified a problem and fleshed it out using the ACT SP/SR five-part problem formulation, you will be able to develop a concise problem statement. Your statement should summarize the problem and include each of the five aspects of problem formulation. See Joann's example on the following page.

EXAMPLE: Joann's Problem Statement

When I think about my breast cancer, I can feel fused with shame, depression, and anxiety. A major component of this is thinking that I know some of my lifestyle can increase the risk of cancer, and I didn't take good enough care of myself. This in turn leads to my wanting to make sure no one in my life is burdened by my self-imposed condition, which leads to social isolation and not allowing others to know how I'm really feeling about my cancer.

EXERCISE. My Problem Statement

Self-Reflective Questions

What was your experience of completing these self-practice exercises? Were these exercises challenging in any way? What came up for you as you completed these exercises?

_____

_____

_____

_____

_____

_____

_____

_____

_____

_____

_____

_____

Did you find it easy or difficult to identify a challenging problem? If you chose a personal problem, did you notice any resistance to searching for an issue there?

_____

_____

_____

_____

_____

_____

_____

_____

_____

_____

_____

How did your completion of these exercises, including an assessment of your current flexibility and emotional experiences, affect the way you experience this problem? How did the exercises in this module affect your experience of yourself in relation to this problem?

_____

_____

_____

_____

_____

_____

_____

_____

_____

_____

_____

_____

Did you notice anything about this problem formulation that is relevant to your clinical practice? What would be useful to reflect on over the next week, in terms of your clinical work? What way of being and doing in relation to practice occur to you here and now?

_____

_____

_____

_____

_____

_____

_____

_____

_____

_____

The Psychological Flexibility Model

ACT interventions aim to help us to develop greater "psychological flexibility" in the service of living lives of meaning, purpose, and vitality. Psychological flexibility can be defined as contacting the present moment fully as a conscious human being, and based on what the situation affords, changing or persisting in behavior in the service of chosen values (Hayes et al., 1999; Kashdan & Rottenberg, 2010). As poetic or aspirational as this definition may sound, it is actually a map of the active process ingredients that we will use in our ACT SP/SR work together. Indeed, when we unpack this definition, we can find a series of specific processes that can be trained through evidence-based techniques (Hayes et al., 2012; Ruiz, 2010).

The psychological flexibility model can be conceptually separated into three aspects of well-being, which are the "three pillars of ACT" that we discussed in Chapter 1. These three dimensions of being open, centered, and engaged, in turn, can be better understood as involving six interacting processes known as:

1. Acceptance (open)
2. Defusion (open)
3. Contacting the present moment (centered)
4. Self-as-context (centered)
5. Values authorship (engaged)
6. Committed action (engaged)

Figure M3.1 illustrates these six processes and how they can be divided into the three pillars of ACT. When we arrange the six processes into a visual illustration such as this, the entire model is known as "the hexaflex." ACT practitioners typically become well versed in this model, training themselves to deliberately target any of these processes in a therapy session or through SP methods. Moving between these processes moment to moment in the flow of a therapy session has even become known as "dancing around the hexaflex" in the ACT community. This flow between the different processes of psychological flexibility is illustrated in Figure M3.1 by the connecting "star-shaped"

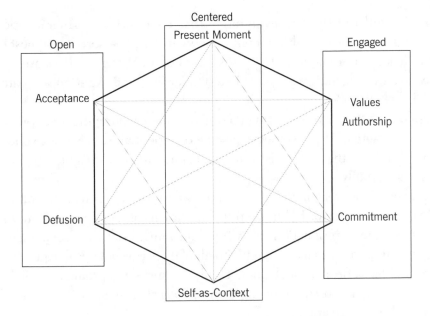

FIGURE 3.1. The hexaflex and the three pillars of ACT.

lines within the hexaflex. In this module, we introduce each of the hexaflex processes and engage with basic experiential practice examples for each.

Acceptance

As the first component of being "open" (and literally the first word in the name of this therapy), acceptance is truly a foundational component of ACT and psychological flexibility. We can imagine acceptance to be "the antidote" to the central problem we target through ACT work: EA (Hayes et al., 1996). EA is a potentially pathological process (Kashdan, Barrios, Forsyth, & Steger, 2006), well known in the psychological literature, involving avoidance and escape of private experiences the individual perceives as aversive. EA becomes pathological when it comes to dominate a person's behavioral repertoires, and when it blocks the individual's pursuit of important endeavors. For example, suppose it's vitally important to a therapist to help their clients learn to live life well. Furthermore, imagine that a therapist accepts a client for therapy who makes them intensely uncomfortable for personal reasons. Perhaps this client vaguely reminds the therapist of a relative who was abusive to the therapist early in life. When the client tells their story, anxiety and shame arise in the therapist. Consequently, the therapist begins to avoid/escape their discomfort by not engaging the client in ways that are important to therapeutic progress. Rather than facing difficult emotions in the therapy session, the therapist distracts the flow of conversation into small talk or supportive "cheerleading." The client might even feel validated by this, but isn't as likely to make significant therapeutic progress. At this point, the avoidance of the therapist's uncomfortable private experience is regulating their behavior rather than the priorities for therapeutic growth. This is not unique to the consulting room. Indeed, living life assertively almost certainly entails psychological discomfort of all sorts for all of us. When our lives are defined by obedience to an EA agenda, we tend to live smaller lives and experience greater suffering (Kashdan et al., 2006).

Acceptance, then, involves letting go of EA while encouraging an approach orientation to valued action. We have devised some experiential exercises for you to pursue later in the workbook that will assist you with coming to know this quality nonverbally, as well as conceptually.

In advance of your reaching that part of the workbook, we provide an initial orientation to this process with words, but keep the limitations of these words in mind. Acceptance does not mean resignation or "white-knuckling." Rather, acceptance involves allowing oneself to freely make contact with all of one's psychological experiences without escape and has a flexible "feel" to it. Think of a surfer who stands on the board rigidly versus one who is loose and dynamic on the board. The latter is an example of the flexibility quality we are after.

✏️ EXERCISE. Self-Practice with Acceptance

Find a quiet place where you will be uninterrupted for about 5–10 minutes for this practice. If you have an area set aside for mindfulness practice, or some quiet time in your office, these contexts will suit the practice well. You can download an audio version of this practice from the book's website (see the box at the end of the table of contents), or record yourself reading the instructions and play them back.

Before you listen to the recording, identify a distressing circumstance related to the problem you are working with in the ACT SP/SR program. As you begin your SP/SR work, it's preferable to select something that's distressful at a 3–4 or less on a 1–10 scale (where 10 = most distressful). This is not because we think private experiences you'd rate higher, say at a 10, are dangerous (because we don't), but rather because when first practicing you are more likely to be successful with something moderately stressful. Imagine you were trying to develop strong swimming strokes, but quickly progressed into deep and rapidly moving water. The tendency there would be to abandon proper body mechanics and just work to survive—that is, you'd be placing yourself in a context that would not pull for the type of learning you are looking for. For analogous reasons we want you to select a context that will help you learn what we mean by acceptance. If you select a circumstance you rate lower than a 5, it may not be sufficiently distressing enough to produce valuable learning either.

Get in a comfortable position in a chair, close your eyes, and bring to mind a recent distressing circumstance related to the problem you have formulated. Once you've selected a circumstance and have begun to imagine it, try to produce the type of psychological struggle you typically experience with this circumstance. You might facilitate this by going through all of your senses in your imagery. See what is there to be seen. Hear any sounds that are there. Feel any sensations that are there. Remain in contact with this struggle against the experience for the next

30 seconds. Now, as you are in contact with the experience, remembering the circumstance, simply sit, openly, in the presence of the totality of your psychological experience. As much as you can, drop the struggle and just allow everything to be there. Notice the physical sensations, emotions, thoughts, and images that move through you as you are in contact with the idea of this challenging situation. As much as you can, remain in this open and receiving mode for the next 30 seconds. Observe what is happening for you, here and now. After these 30 seconds of full acceptance, again return to struggling against your experience in the way that you typically might. Whatever ways you might use to distract yourself, redirect your attention, block, or resist contacting your experience of this painful circumstance, this is your time to use them with freedom and abandon. Go ahead and indulge your EA. After 30 seconds, allow yourself three mindful breaths, and return to an open and receiving mode of experience. As much as you can, be fully with whatever arises, here and now. Alternate back and forth a few times between struggle and open acceptance until you feel you've gotten a "taste" of allowing yourself to make contact with your private experiences without fighting the experiences themselves. Notice the contrast between the open orientation and attempts to push away your experience. After a few iterations, again allow yourself three deep and cleansing mindful breaths. When you are ready, open your eyes and return your attention to the room around you and to our work together in this workbook.

After you've completed this exercise, write down some reflections and observations of your experience of direct engagement with acceptance below.

Defusion

The second component of the "open" dimension of psychological flexibility, "defusion," is best understood by first understanding its pathological opposite: fusion. In essence, the term *cognitive fusion* (Blackledge, 2007) refers to the process whereby words and cognitions come to dominate the regulation of our behavior by overpowering the influence of our direct experience of the world. As we discussed, this occurs as we experience thoughts and words as if they literally *were* the things to which they refer, rather than symbols. In such cases, our behaviors are predicted and influenced by imaginal stimuli as if they were actual events in the world, rather than events in the mind. For example, even if you were in a dark room and having thoughts about the sun, or memories of enjoyable times sunbathing, a number of literalized functions may become psychologically present. In your imagination, you may experience warmth, brightness, a round object, or the color yellow. If you were sufficiently absorbed by these mental events involving the sun the way we might be during ruminations, daydreams, or when "haunted" by a memory, you might even lose sight of the fact that the sun is not literally present.

Another way to understand this process is to examine what a belief really is. What do we mean when we refer to a "belief"? Really think about this before you read on. Typically, we might mean to believe something to be true, so we imagine that our representation of a thing accords with what is happening in the outside world, or "reality." For example, if I say that I believe that my hometown is a good place to live, you might assume that this means that there is an existing town in an objective reality that is "good" for me. A contextual behavioral science and ACT-consistent perspective is not so interested in whether a belief corresponds with a potential objective "reality." We are much more interested in how our "beliefs," as mental events and private behaviors, influence and predict our subsequent actions. Does this mental event lead to workable actions? How does my having the mental representation of my town as "good" influence my decisions and movement toward valued aims? Does it make my life smaller or bigger?

In this way, our perspective is that a "belief" is really a proxy variable for a thought–action relationship. When a person says they "believe" something, that person is essentially saying that they are going to act on the basis of the word's literal meaning. For example, when a client says they believe that they are "unlovable," the client is saying that their behavior is largely regulated by the literal meaning of those words. The client is saying that they will "act on the basis of" this idea. Fusion happens when the literal functions of words come to regulate behavior and other available functions become irrelevant.

Defusion, then, is the process by which the dominance of one function (i.e., the literal function) over other available functions is reduced. When we train our mind to experience thoughts as thoughts, facilitating a *transformation of stimulus functions* so that we are no longer tyrannized by the beliefs, thoughts, and images that go through our mind, we are practicing defusion. When we are able to view mental events as what they are, rather than what they appear to be, we are able to reclaim our course of action in our lives through defusion.

EXERCISE. Self-Practice with Defusion

As we begin experiencing defusion from the inside out, let's learn it the way many of our clients may have first experienced defusion practice in session. The classic ACT "Milk, Milk, Milk" (Hayes et al., 1999) exercise has served as the introductory defusion technique for thousands of clients throughout the world over the last decades. Beyond that, the original exercise dates from practices used by Titchener (1916) over a century ago. In ACT, we have adapted Titchener's original word repetition experiments as a clinical intervention, but the core of the practice remains the same. So, as we begin our defusion work, we are definitely going "old school."

To begin the practice, say "milk" out loud and notice what shows up psychologically. Go ahead, do this now. We'll wait. What did you notice? An image of milk in a glass or a carton? A cow? Perhaps you remembered pouring cold milk on some crisp cereal and listening to the crackle of your breakfast. Next, use the timer app on your phone or a watch with a second hand and prepare to time a 45-second period. You will repeat the word *milk* rapidly for 45 seconds out loud. When ready, begin, and say "milk" repeatedly as quickly as you can for 45 seconds.

What did you notice popping into your head related to milk as you were repeatedly saying the word? What are you thinking now? Did anything happen to those psychological events that were present for you just a little while ago—that is, did anything happen to the image of the glass, carton, or cow? Did you start to experience different things with this word when it was repeated? Perhaps the word became difficult to say or sounded like a funny sound. This happened because repeating the word rapidly stripped the word of its literal meaning functions and allowed some of the other functions to become more dominant, such as the auditory functions. The functions changed through repetition, through experience of a word in a new and strange context.

Now, pick a thought that is related to the problem area that you chose, and repeat the exercise. For example, if you struggled with the thought "I'm a bad parent," you would say this sentence out loud and would notice what became psychologically present for you. Next, you would get your timing device and would repeat "I'm a bad parent" over and over as quickly as you could, even when it became difficult to say, for 45 seconds. Next, you would notice what happened to those psychological events, thoughts, and images. Would they still be present in the same way? What other functions would become present? Choose a sentence from your problem area for this exercise.

> Write your observations of what you noticed while experiencing the "Milk, Milk, Milk" exercise and while repeating a phrase from your problem area below.

Contacting the Present Moment

The first process involved in the "centered" dimension of the psychological flexibility model represents our ability to contact the present moment and all that it contains. This means that our ability to attend to what is arising in our awareness, moment by moment, with a focus on the immediate experience of now, is an important part of our capacity to adaptively respond to our environment and live well. Wisdom traditions have prioritized training present-moment-focused awareness for thousands of years. Indeed, the ability to attend in the moment is at the heart of mindfulness, concentration, and attention training in Buddhist psychology (Tirch, Silberstein, & Kolts, 2015). However, this capacity isn't always as available as we may think it is. Throughout the course of our days, our attention isn't often solely "in the present." Rather, our attention is often "in the past" (like when we depressively ruminate) or "in the future" (like when we're anxious and engage in "What if?"–type activity). This creates a number of difficulties, most notable of which is that we cannot optimally track moment-by-moment changes in the contingencies governing our behavior under these conditions. This type of unfocused and inflexible attention often blocks us from choosing response options that would make us more effective in our lives.

Cultivating our ability to contact the present moment involves enhancing the attentional control skill of attending to events in the present, nonjudgmentally and voluntarily. It is the core skill in the ACT conceptualization of mindfulness and it can be trained through specific practices. The exercise below will be familiar to you, in some variation. In fact, this practice is an iteration of the earlier centering exercise we provided, with a gradually greater emphasis on contacting your present-moment experience. We invite you to encounter the practice, as if for the first time, and as it relates to your engagement with your problem area chosen for SP/SR work.

EXERCISE. Self-Practice Contacting the Present Moment

Allow a good 10 minutes in a quiet and comfortable space for this practice. If you practice the exercise in silence, it is a good idea to set a timer so that you do not "eyeball" the time duration during your practice period. You may benefit most from this exercise if you read the script into a recording device so that you can listen to it and simply follow the instructions, or you can download the audio version of this practice from the book's website (see the box at the end of the table of contents).

Close your eyes and allow your breathing to descend into a natural, balanced rhythm. Bring to mind the problem area and spend a few moments just breathing in the presence of the thoughts, emotions, and physical sensations that arise in awareness after reminding yourself of the problem. [pause] You don't need to specifically focus on thoughts about the problem. Just allow the mind to be wherever it is as you begin. [pause] During this time, part of our attention is in the breath, observing the inbreath and the outbreath. As much as you can, allow your attention to rest on the flow of the breath, in and out of the body. [pause] Notice the rhythm of your breathing. There's no need for you to artificially increase or decrease the pace of your breathing. Just simply let it settle into the pace of its choosing. Now, begin to observe the path that the air takes as you breathe in and out. [pause] That is, watch the path that the air takes as it goes in through your nose, down your lungs, and in and out of your belly. Just observe this. When your mind wanders, as it will certainly do, just notice that it has wandered and gently bring awareness, again, back to your breath. Don't fight to bring it back. Just notice where your awareness goes and then gently and tenderly bring it back to your breath. [pause] After a few moments, see whether you can notice, nonjudgmentally, the sensation the air makes as it brushes against your nostrils. Just notice this sensation. [pause] See whether you can notice the temperature of the air as it comes in and out of your nose. Is it warm? [pause] Cool? [pause] Finally, see whether you can notice how long the sensation of the air brushing up against your nostrils lingers after your outbreath. How long can you detect even the faintest sensation? Forming an intention to let go of this exercise, begin to gradually return your awareness to your surroundings, gently opening your eyes, and bringing your attention back into the room.

When the alarm sounds to indicate the completion of this exercise, or the audio is complete, provide some reflections on this experience in the space below.

Self-as-Context

The second component of being "centered" in ACT is described as an experience of "self-as-context." This dimension of psychological flexibility refers to a perspective that goes beyond our conventional conceptualized sense of ourself as an individual living through a personal narrative. Our ability to experience ourself as an observer of our experience is what we point to when we discuss self-as-context. Many meditation and wisdom traditions have written on the experience of a transcendent sense of self for centuries (Deikman, 1982). In the contemplative practice literature, we can find many references to meditators abiding as pure awareness, observing their moment-by-moment experience with equanimity, and dis-identifying from any of their narrative self-experience. This robust human capacity for flexible perspective taking and a transcendent sense of self is a foundational part of personal transformation through ACT SP/SR.

ACT therapists speak of three senses of self: the conceptualized self, self-as-ongoing awareness, and self-as-context (Barnes-Holmes, Hayes, & Dymond, 2001). If we were to ask you to provide as many responses as you could to the sentence stem "I am a person who _____," you would likely readily generate many descriptions such as "is tall," "is trying my best," "is female," "is old," "is likable," "is outgoing," and so on. These descriptions form the basis of the conceptualized self. From childhood we are taught to use verbal descriptions to categorize and define our behavior and our self-experience. That is a part of the universal human experience. Over time, because of the relational activity of the mind, we come to string these descriptions together into a story and then we begin to respond to the story as if it were an absolute reality, with the narrative exerting supreme influence. In this sense, our conceptualized sense of self causes us to respond in narrow and inflexible ways that interrupt our ability to live well.

Self-as-ongoing awareness, the second sense of self articulated in ACT, involves our previously discussed capacity to fully contact the present moment. During present-moment contact, we have the opportunity to self-experience in a defused and accepting way. We notice the flow of our experience, and we simply attend, moment by moment, as events arise. This sense of self-experience is sometimes referred to as a "self-as-process" mode of being, as we are actively attending to the processes arising in our mind. As we experience the "I/here/nowness" (Hayes et al., 2012) of being through contacting our ongoing, present-focused awareness, we create the conditions necessary to shift into an awareness of ourselves as a flexible perspective that facilitates an "observing self" experience. Our sense of being a separate self can fade from awareness as we experience a deepening interiority and spacious ground of being. Self-as-context involves taking a perspective of our private events. It involves becoming aware of the location from which we "observe" our psychological activity.

EXERCISE. Self-Practice with Self-as-Context

For this practice, again find a quiet space where you will not be disturbed for at least 10 minutes. We are going to repeat a variation on the contacting the present moment exercise we asked you to practice earlier. Use a self-recording of the instructions below or download an audio version of this practice from the book's website (see the box at the end of the table of contents). We are again connecting with the present moment, but will broaden and deepen our perspective to more fully become aware of our awareness itself through this practice.

Close your eyes and allow your breathing to descend into a natural, balanced rhythm. Spend a few moments just breathing in the presence of the thoughts, emotions, and physical sensations that arise in awareness after reminding yourself of the problem. [pause] *You don't need to specifically focus on thoughts about the problem. Just allow the mind to be wherever it is as you begin.* [pause] *During this time, part of our attention is in the breath, observing the inbreath and the outbreath. As much as you can, allow your attention to rest on the flow of the breath, in and out of the body.* [pause] *Notice the rhythm of your breathing. There's no need for you to artificially increase or decrease the pace of your breathing. Just simply let it settle into the pace of its choosing. Now, begin to observe the path that the air takes as you breathe in and out.* [pause] *That is, watch the path that the air takes as it goes in through your nose, down your lungs, and in and out of your belly. Just observe this. When your mind wanders, as it will certainly do, just notice that it has wandered and gently bring awareness, again, back to your breath. Don't fight to bring it back. Just notice where your awareness goes and then gently and tenderly bring it back to your breath.* [pause] *After a few moments, see whether you can notice, nonjudgmentally, the sensation the air makes as it brushes against your nostrils. Just notice this sensation.* [pause] *See whether you can notice the temperature of the air as it comes in and out of your nose. Is it warm?* [pause] *Cool?* [pause] *See whether you can notice how long the sensation of the air brushing up against your nostrils lingers after your outbreath. How long can you detect even the faintest sensation?*

Now, notice the part of you that is watching your breath. We notice our breath. [long pause] *We notice our awareness of our breath.* [long pause] *We notice our awareness of our awareness.* [long pause] *Breathing in, and breathing out, connecting with yourself as pure awareness. Breathing in, I am aware of my awareness of my breath.* [long pause] *Breathing out, I am aware of my awareness. I am aware of my awareness.* [pause] *I am awareness. I am awareness.* [pause] *I am.* [pause] *I am.* [pause] *And whatever is showing up for you, here and now, it is OK for you to experience it. Allow. It's OK if you only briefly catch a glimpse. It's OK. You are here and now. If you have an evaluation of your practice such as "I'm not doing this right!" see whether you can catch, even if only briefly, the part of yourself that is watching and aware of that thought. Don't persist with this too long. The point is not to master this skill. The point is to make initial experiential contact with this process. We'll have more in-depth exercises for you later in this workbook. Forming an intention to let go of this exercise, begin to gradually return your awareness to your surroundings, gently opening your eyes, and bringing your attention back into the room.*

When the alarm sounds to indicate the completion of this exercise, or the audio is complete, provide some reflections on this experience in the space below.

Values Authorship

In ACT, the first dimension of being "engaged" in life is described as "values" author-ship. Values are described as freely chosen, verbally constructed qualities of doing and being that establish a sense of meaning, purpose, and vitality in our lives. Indeed, ACT therapists sometimes describe values as "vital directions." Values are *vital* because they are of central importance to our lives, and they are *directions* because there is no pos-sibility of final arrival. For example, as a therapist you may value reducing psychological suffering of your clients, and value helping them to enhance meaning in their lives. Let's notice that this kind of work can never be truly complete and finished. As long as you are healthy and functional, you can always reduce more suffering and help more clients. Your work is a lifelong pursuit. In a similar fashion, values are best thought of as verbs rather than nouns. So, when we imagine that you value reducing client suffering, we are referring to the way you choose to behave rather than the way you feel inside. The central emphasis in ACT is in increasing values-based living, because the bottom line is that if it's not in your behavior, then it's not in your life.

Values should be discriminated from goals. Values are endless, whereas goals are finite. Goals are important because they motivate valued behavior and because they are indicative of values-congruent living. For instance, you may help a client get unstuck during a course of therapy and then collaboratively decide to terminate with the client. The termination is an objective endpoint that is an element of a larger pattern of your behavior that we might label "reducing client suffering and enhancing meaning." Fur-thermore, as soon as we set an intention and begin to move toward realizing our values, our values are already in motion. For example, if I told you that I had a "goal" to walk downtown to a shop, my realization of that goal would take place when I reached the shop and stepped inside. However, if I have a "value" of "heading south," as soon as I begin to move my foot in that direction, I am already manifesting my valued aim. ACT therapists have a range of methods for working with values authorship, and research has demonstrated that working with values can play a large part in successful client outcomes (Wilson & Murrell, 2004).

✍️ EXERCISE. Self-Practice with Values Authorship

The Imaginary Eulogy is a classic, ACT-consistent experiential practice for reflection on values authorship. Variations on this metaphorical exercise can be found in 12-step work, modern CBT, and ACT practice (Hayes, 2005; Hayes et al., 2012). It serves well as an introductory practice for engaging with the construction of our valued aims. The instructions for the practice are provided below in transcript form, and the audio of the exercise is available on the book's website (see the box at the end of the table of contents). The practice guides us through imagining what attending our own funeral and hearing our eulogy might be like. We are invited to imagine two versions of this eulogy. The first would be the one we might hear if we were to carry on with our lives with business as usual, without making any major changes in our behavior. The second version of the eulogy represents what we might hear if we were to intentionally live our lives in accordance with our most heartfelt values. This exercise invites us to ask ourselves "What do I want my life to stand for?" and "What do I want my legacy to be?"

As you begin, allow your eyes to close. Begin to focus on your breathing. Settle your awareness on the level of physical sensation, allowing your attention to gather on the breath. Allow each inbreath and outbreath to flow in its own rhythm. Beyond this, allow yourself to inhabit this awareness, abiding in a state of bare observation, suspending judgment, or evaluation, or even description. Your mind may wander away from the breath, away from this exercise, and if this happens, simply notice the wandering mind and gently return your attention to this practice.

On the next inbreath, begin to imagine that it is 10 years from now and you have won an all-expenses-paid trip to a remote tropical destination, and en route your plane has to make an emergency crash landing and you find yourself stranded. You and your fellow travelers are all safe—however, you are cut off from civilization. Back home, your friends and family are told of the accident and that you have died. Unaware of your survival, they begin to plan your funeral. In the meantime, after a week on the island, you are saved by a passing fishing boat that unfortunately does not have a working radio. The day you return home happens to be the day of your funeral. You arrive at the funeral moments before your eulogy. Standing at the back of the crowd you go unnoticed and listen as your loved ones speak about your life, what was meaningful to you, about you, what you will be remembered for. You listen to their words and look around at those who are dear to you. Who is there? Who is speaking? What do they say?

Sit with this experience for a few moments and exploring what your loved ones would say if you had continued to live your life, including these last 10 years on autopilot, trapped by old habits and struggles with thoughts and emotions—finding yourself on a path that moved you away from what was most important to you.

After spending some time with this, on the next available outbreath, let go of this part of the exercise and with the inbreath gently return your attention to mindful breathing. Noticing the rise and fall of the abdomen as you breathe in and breathe out.

Now, with the next inbreath, begin to imagine that you have arrived to this funeral after having lived your life, and especially the last 10 years embodying your most cherished values and in a manner that reflected your meaning and purpose. Once again, imagine yourself standing at the back of your funeral service, unnoticed and listening as your loved ones speak about you and about your life. As you imagine those people at your funeral, who is in attendance? Imagine yourself watching them listening to your eulogy. And who is speaking? What are people saying about those things you said and did? What are people remembering you for?

Allow yourself to sit with this experience for a few moments and consider what your loved ones would say if you had made changes in your life and choices that filled you with purpose and vitality. That you took a path of valued living, engaged with those people, places, and activities that mean the most to you.

After spending some time with this experience, when you are ready and on the next available outbreath, let go of this imagery and with the inbreath gently return your attention to mindful breathing. Noticing the rise and fall of the abdomen as you breathe in and breathe out. Now, with the next inbreath, allow your attention to focus on the sounds that surround you in the room. Next, bring the attention to the sounds outside of the room. Following this, allow your attention to gently settle on the sounds even farther away than that. Giving yourself a few moments to gather your attention and orientation to your presence in your chair, and when you feel ready, you can open your eyes.

When your practice is complete, provide some reflections on this experience in the space below.

Committed Action

Committed action is as central to practicing ACT as it is to the name of the therapy. Committed action is the ultimate psychological flexibility process we are introducing, and in many ways it is the ultimate aim of the therapy itself. The second aspect of the "engaged" pillar of the hexaflex, committed action describes a pattern of behavior that exemplifies the realization of our heart's deepest desires for how we wish to be in the world.

The "commitment" in committed action represents more than just making a promise to behave in a certain way (Hayes et al., 2012). In fact, the specific way that we approach commitment in ACT involves how we respond in the present moment, and has certain defined characteristics. When we make a commitment toward a behavior in the service of our valued aims, we are, essentially, making a decision in advance. We are taking a private experience, such as thinking about taking action, and we are making this a public experience by committing to take such actions verbally with another person, or in writing. This moves our valued aim outside of the realm of our mental experiences and begins to bring our potential actions into the realm of the actual. Research suggests that commitments we make publicly and with specificity are more likely to result in effective action than commitments that we consider only in our own mind. Also, commitment does not mean inflexibly following a behavior plan without any deviation. Committed action entails the important feature of continuously redirecting one's behavior toward what's important, rather than away from what's present and aversive in each moment, and gradually constructing larger patterns of behavior of this type. A large part of commitment and valued living involves returning again and again to pursuing our valued aims, when we have made mistakes or have lost our way.

✍️ EXERCISE. Self-Practice with Committed Action

Earlier in this module we used an imaginary eulogy practice to help you imagine what it would be like to realize your values and live your life as the version of yourself that you most wish to be. Now, we are going to experientially touch upon what it means to fully commit to realizing that vision. Although all six processes in the psychological flexibility model are interlinked, perhaps values and committed action are more connected with each other than any of the other four. Values are to highways as committed action is to cars. Once we know what highway we want to get on, we now have to drive the car. Driving the car, however, entails confronting obstacles. We will experience congested traffic, construction, and detours. We will make use of the other processes to negotiate these obstacles, bringing everything together.

Allow a good 5–10 minutes in a quiet location for this exercise. As with the previous eyes-closed exercises, we recommend that you record this script and listen to it in a contemplative setting, or download the audio version of this practice from the book's website (see the box at the end of the table of contents).

When you're ready, find a comfortable and grounded position in your chair, and spend the next 30 seconds or so gathering your attention and practicing being present. Gently placing your attention on the parts of your body that are making contact with the place where you are sitting. Feel the support of the floor, the seat of the chair, and your presence here and now. Take a few mindful breaths and orient yourself to our practice.

Bring to mind an important valued aim you have that relates to the problem area you have identified. In ACT, we sometimes say, "In your pain you can find your values, and in your values, you can find your pain." Inside this problem there is something that matters deeply to you. What is it that you care about that is involved in this problem area? Bring that to mind and spend the next minute reflecting on the core value that is related to this difficulty.

Now, let's identify one goal that is related to this valued aim. Let's bring to mind a goal that is small and very manageable. What is one thing, no matter how small, that you could do that could make a difference in bringing you a bit further toward this valued aim? Even a small goal like this might be challenging for you, and may be likely to bring up some discomfort. Perhaps it's associated with boredom or fear. Maybe it stirs up some sadness. For example, if I wanted to quit smoking for the rest of my life, and I set an aim to go even just one morning without smoking any cigarettes, that might be a challenge, might it not? Let's frame an idea of one small step that you can commit to here and now, in this workbook, that will move you toward something that matters. If you wanted to reorganize your entire home, you could commit to cleaning and rearranging one shelf of cups or dishes. Remember that moving toward our values takes place inside every step. The main thing here for us is that you can identify and commit to one thing. With this small step you can make a true decision, a creative decision—and true and creative decisions, followed by committed action, can change our world. Imagine yourself behaving toward this goal, and taking this small step. Visualize your success in this small step.

Write and describe the small step toward living your values that you have chosen.

My small step toward a valued aim is:

Do I commit to taking action toward realizing this goal?

When your practice is complete, provide some reflections on this experience in the space below.

Self-Reflective Questions

What was your experience as you engaged in the core elements of psychological flexibility experientially?

_____

_____

_____

_____

_____

_____

_____

_____

_____

_____

_____

_____

_____

You may be familiar with these concepts and practices, but perhaps this is a new way to engage with them. What did you learn about psychological flexibility from this way of working?

_____

_____

_____

_____

_____

_____

_____

_____

_____

_____

_____

_____

What did you notice about how psychological flexibility relates to the problem that you are dealing with through your ACT SP/SR work?

_____

_____

_____

_____

_____

_____

_____

_____

_____

_____

_____

_____

Are there new elements of this problem that you are now able to see? How might approaching the problem by cultivating psychological flexibility differ from "problem solving"?

_____

_____

_____

_____

_____

_____

_____

_____

_____

_____

_____

_____

_____

From your experience, what would it be like to bring greater psychological flexibility in your psychotherapy work? How would your work be different? What would it look like?

_____

_____

_____

_____

_____

_____

_____

_____

_____

_____

_____

_____

_____

From your experience, how does psychological flexibility relate to directly pursuing your values in clinical work? In what ways might the opposite of psychological flexibility be holding you back as a clinician?

_____

_____

_____

_____

_____

_____

_____

_____

_____

_____

_____

_____

The ACT Matrix

As we proceed with our ACT SP/SR program, we continually clarify our valued aims and intentions, and deepen our engagement with psychological flexibility. As you have seen, ACT SP/SR begins in a similar fashion to that of clinical ACT work by establishing some baseline measures, getting a sense of valued aims, and orienting to the processes involved in ACT. ACT is an experiential mode of psychotherapy, and each step of our work is designed to experientially move the core process involved in realizing our human potential. In this way, every step of our ACT SP/SR is the work itself, and nothing is "preparatory" or "theoretical." This next module is intended to help you build a stronger foundation for realizing your intention and action. To do this, we use the deceptively simple "matrix" diagram that is widely utilized in ACT practice.

The matrix diagram is a clinical and supervisory tool used in ACT that can help orient individuals toward psychological flexibility and its related processes. It can serve both as a case conceptualization tool and an intervention in and of itself (Polk, 2014; Schoendorff, Webster, & Polk, 2014). In fact, some ACT therapists make working with the matrix the major, if not sole, focus of their technical base, to great effect. The matrix is intended to help individuals and groups (1) notice their experiences and (2) manifest meaningful and purposeful ways of embodying their values through committed action.

The matrix was designed to simplify ACT work and to enable brief, direct interventions. As such, the matrix is just a very simple diagram of two perpendicular lines, one vertical and one horizontal. Just like x and y axes in a geometry class or math text, the matrix represents a simple cross on a page, as we see below.

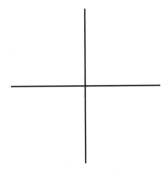

As the lines intersect, they create four quadrants in the visual space or sheet of paper on which they are drawn. It is remarkable how much human behavior can be guided by simply drawing a cross and giving people a few instructions. Interestingly, working with a tetrad to guide problem conceptualization predates ACT work, and can be found in the systematics work of John G. Bennett (*www.systematics.org/journal/vol1-1/GeneralSystematics.htm*)—some form of this dates as far back as Pythagoras. However, our ACT matrix tool developed independent of these lines of thought, and is grounded in an aim to simplify ACT work for brief interventions (Polk, 2014).

When we use the matrix, we explain to our clients that we write down things that happen in our lives on a sheet of paper and then sort these experiences into the four quadrants created by drawing these lines. In this way, each quadrant in the matrix represents a domain of human experience. The two quadrants above the horizontal (x) axis represent observable behaviors and actions that take place in the outside world. These are observable behaviors and actions that can be seen by anyone present. For example, driving to work, doing the laundry, or eating a piece of cake would be observable and would be considered events in the "outside word." Such events would be sorted into the top two quadrants of the matrix. In turn, the two quadrants below the horizontal axis line represent mental events. These are the thoughts, emotions, and imaginings that might be described as taking place in the "inside world." In behaviorist language, the overt behaviors that are described in the top half of the diagram are called "public events," as they can be viewed and known by more than one person. The covert behaviors that are described in the lower half of the diagram are known as "private events" because such mental events are accessible only to the experiencer themselves.

Taking a look at the vertical division at the center of the matrix, we can see the page divided into two sections, left and right. All of the space in the two quadrants to the left of the center represents experiences and actions that involve attempts to avoid or move away from our direct experience. This half of the matrix is known as the "away" half because events that we write into this quadrant involve moving away from our experiencing. Events and experiences that are sorted and written down in the right-hand half of the matrix are events that move us closer to our valued aims. Accordingly, the right-hand half of the matrix is known as the "toward" section of the diagram. The illustration on the next page provides a more detailed description of these sections of the matrix, and of how we work with this clinical tool in ACT SP/SR.

Experienced in the Outside World

My Identified Avoidant Patterns of Action	My "Toward Moves": My values-focused practices and habits
My Hooks: What unwanted thoughts and feelings might get in the way?	**My Values: What qualities of doing, being, and relating matter most to me?**

Mental Events

When we work with the matrix, we often begin with the bottom right quadrant, asking our clients what they value most in their lives. From the lower right, we can move clockwise through the remaining four quadrants, examining those actions and mental events that result in a struggle with painful experiences, as opposed to behaviors and practices that move an individual toward their deepest valued aims.

The matrix is an active and engaging tool that brings the core processes of ACT to life for the individual and allows for effective choice and clarification of individualized aims (Schoendorff et al., 2014). Now, we walk through the processes in the matrix and use an ACT SP/SR matrix tool to help you work with the problem area you have chosen for this workbook.

Processes in the Matrix

Taking the Position of the Observer:
"You Are the Experiencer, Not the Experience."

At the center of the matrix diagram there is a circle indicating the process of observing your experience, sometimes described as "me noticing the difference." This is the central practice in the matrix, noticing your experience of where you are at this moment in space and time, and noticing where you are focusing your attention (Schoendorff et al., 2014). We all move through the world with varying levels of attention and awareness on our inner and outer experiences. For example, sometimes we are focused on our internal experiences, such as thoughts or how we are feeling physically, while at other times we are more attuned to our experience of the outside world and what is unfolding around us. Using the matrix provides us with an opportunity to get to know our observer self and to sharpen our ability to notice and discriminate between our experiences.

Discriminating between Private and Public Experiences

When we use the matrix, we practice discriminating between mental experiencing and five-senses experiencing (Polk, 2014). This is also known as private experiencing and public experiencing. As we have seen, increasing our freedom to pursue our valued aims while becoming less controlled by our responses to mental formations is a central focus of ACT. Discriminating between mental events and contingencies in the actual world is a deceptively subtle skill that is necessary in this process.

One way to understand this process of noticing these two classes of experience is to pick up an object within reach, perhaps even this book, or the electronic device you may be using to read these words. Take a moment to observe and notice this physical object. Using some of your five senses, what do you experience? What does it look like? What does it smell like? When you flip through or close the book, what sounds do you hear? Next, put the book away, out of the reach of your five senses, and allow yourself to imagine the experience of a book. See whether you can recall what the book looks like. What it felt like in your hands. See whether you can re-create this experience in your mind. Notice the mental experience of the book. Do you notice a difference between these two experiences? The first is what you experience in an interaction with the outside world, what you can observe with the five senses. The second is what you experience in your private world, as mental representations of the world.

In this way, attending to public or sensory experiencing includes responding to our observable behaviors and what we hear, touch, taste, smell, and see. Our private experiencing includes mental events, such as thoughts, images, and memories, as well as emotions, urges, and sensations. Physical sensations are considered private events or inner experiencing in using the matrix because they often occur on the inside of our skin and body (Polk, 2014). As we see next, this discrimination between mind and matter is useful in identifying what private experiences get in the way of our realizing our values, and what behaviors we engage in to avoid unwanted experiences.

Discriminating between "Toward" and "Away" Experiences

The matrix also asks us to discriminate between experiences that involve movement toward valued directions versus experiences that involve movement away from unwanted experiences. To get a sense of this process, take a moment to remember what it is like for you when you are engaged in values-driven behaviors. See whether you can recall a time when you were moving toward something that was truly important to you—perhaps, showing up to take care of a friend or a family member, going to a yoga class, or heading out for a run. Notice what moving toward this value was like for you.

Now, remember a time when you struggled with an unwanted private experience or mental event. Perhaps a worrying thought or upsetting image. We all have some anxiety or worry, particularly about the things that we care about. Choose a thought related to your problem area chosen for this workbook. Now that you have that thought in your mind, remember how you struggled with, or tried to avoid, the experience of this difficult thought. Remember what you might have done to get rid of that experience. Do you notice differences between these two experiences of moving toward values versus moving away from unwanted inner experiences? How did you feel when you were engaged in realizing your values? In contrast, how did you feel when you were struggling against your experience? Remember the consequences of these two directions. As we just lightly touched on these discriminations together, we can begin to appreciate how differently these two classes of experience and action affect our being.

Values Authorship in the Matrix

The construction of valued aims is also a part of working with the matrix. In order to notice when someone is moving toward what is important to them, it is necessary to know what is personally meaningful and important, if not essential. In using the ACT matrix, values are understood as private events, in that they are not tangible outcomes but "verbally constructed" (cognitively represented) directions toward what is most important to us. They help shape our valued aims and engage in "toward" moves. When we list "who and what is important" in the lower right quadrant of the matrix, we are really looking for examples of how we wish to be in the world in terms of "who and what is important." For example, one of us (Dennis) struggled with how to balance being present for family on the weekends, while still completing necessary writing and research projects. A few of the items that were recorded in that quadrant, which represented valued aims, were "being a loving and engaged uncle," "spending meaningful time with my partner," "bringing active attention and creativity to my writing," and "spending time exercising." All of these were activities, but in the lower right quadrant of the matrix we record them as visions of how we wish to be in the world, rather than specific practices or goals.

"The Thoughts That Hook You"

The matrix asks us to identify those unwanted inner experiences that cause us to be hooked into recurring patterns of struggle and emotional suffering. This includes any thoughts, emotions, memories, mental images, physical sensations, or urges that might be experienced as barriers to one's values (Polk, 2014). When we list the "unwanted internal stuff" that chronically shows up for us in the lower left quadrant, we are listing those fears, worries, ruminations, and difficult thoughts that seem to drive our suffering. These inner hooks can take many forms, and yet some of them seem all too familiar. For instance, in the example above, Dennis found that his mind would tell him a litany of critical thoughts that often created an inescapable double bind. For example, hooks that were listed in this quadrant included "What kind of a person neglects his family on the weekend? You are a selfish workaholic!" if he was working on a project in his study. However, if he was spending time building a puzzle with his nephew, Dennis's inner critic would tell him, "How can you just waste your time indulging yourself playing when you have work to do? You're pathetically lazy!" As you may notice in the practice to come, the simple act of taking an observing, defused perspective and listing these mental hooks and unwanted private experiences can set the stage for distancing from these thoughts, and getting out from under their excessive influence.

Avoidant Actions

The matrix then asks participants to observe the ways in which they respond to these blocks with observable behaviors in the outside world. As we begin to list these actions in the upper left-hand quadrant, we might ask ourselves what we do to deal with or distract ourselves from unwanted inner experiences. Here, the key process to notice and focus on are those avoidance behaviors that keep us "stuck" in psychologically inflexible approaches. When your blocks show up, what do you usually do in response to them? What avoidant patterns might show up so automatically that we don't even notice them as avoidance? We are looking for those EA behaviors that seem to keep us stuck and prevent moving toward our values and committed actions (Polk, 2014). Some people might drown their sorrows in Pinot Grigio, while others might isolate, engage in compulsive rituals, or procrastinate. The range of avoidant actions is broad, and some seemingly values-based behaviors might be avoidance in disguise. For example, Dennis found that he would inadvertently avoid the distressing conflict between spending time with family or writing by taking up seemingly urgent "busywork" tasks, like reorganizing the office or tuning and repairing a guitar. While drawn into this seemingly important work, he could distract his mind from the values conflict involved in either dedicating time to family or meaningful projects. While the distress would be avoided at first, he was denied the opportunity to deeply engage with the things that mattered most. While cleaning house and fixing musical instruments is usually a better option than binge drinking or hiding from the world, the function of avoidance is the same. In a sense, when we explore and list our avoidance-based behaviors, we are using our understanding of the functional analysis of behavior to choose which practices and habits we want to cultivate, based on whether they make our lives bigger or smaller.

Choosing Valued Behaviors

The matrix diagram is a tool intended to increase one's noticing their experiences and to get unstuck from the struggle with unwanted inner experiencing (Polk, 2015). But in ACT, this is not an end to itself. Ultimately, we wish to generate healthy practices and actions that will increase our committed action in the service of our valued aims through work with the matrix. When we populate the upper right-hand quadrant of the matrix, we are simply listing those directly observable behaviors that will help us move in the direction of the values we listed just below this quadrant. This area will be filled with actions that help us to be the version of ourselves we most wish to be. If we were free from having our behaviors controlled by the "hooks" of our thoughts and feelings in the bottom left, and we could train ourselves to let go of habitual patterns of action in the top left, what would we be doing with our "hands and feet" to "walk the walk" in our everyday lives? For instance, in the example we have been following, Dennis listed several things that served a work–life balance, and created a healthy context for spending time with both academic psychology work and family. He listed things like:

"Maintaining good sleep and wake hygiene."
"Keeping a healthy diet and abstaining from alcohol."
"Waking at 5:30 A.M."
"Beginning the day with a seated Zen meditation and a healthy breakfast."
"Getting 30–60 minutes of exercise each day."
"Writing first thing in the morning for a minimum of an hour."
"Attending to organizational tasks after writing."
"Scheduling time with family and friends on weekend days in specific ways."
"Using unscheduled weekend time for a blend of further writing work and restful recreation."

These steps became habits, and before noon on a weekend day, Dennis typically found that he had engaged in writing, contemplative practice, exercise, and organization in a way that served his valued aims. This left time available to be truly present with family in a loving and connected way. Such behavior changes happened "overnight," but only after years of working hard to deliberately build new practices and habits. Even after building these repertoires, they take time and dedication to maintain, with little failures along the way.

Importantly, let's remember that committed action doesn't mean selecting these new actions once and flawlessly engaging in them without fail. As the pioneering IBM leader Thomas J. Watson famously said, "If you want to increase your success rate, double your failure rate." ACT cofounder Kelly Wilson (Wilson & DuFrene, 2012) has described psychological flexibility with the following poetic question:

> In this very moment, will you accept the sad and the sweet, hold lightly your stories about what is possible, and be the author of a life that has meaning and purpose for you, turning in kindness back to that life when you find yourself moving away from it? (p. 13)

Our key point in using the matrix, and, indeed, in using ACT SP/SR as a whole, is that when we deliberately notice and specify our valued aims, and when we open our eyes to take into account the mental events and behaviors that get in our way, we can more effectively choose to live from a place of wisdom, strength, and commitment by deliberately returning to expanding patterns of valued action that can change our world and extend our values into the world around us.

The Matrix in ACT SP/SR

On the next few pages you will find a blank ACT SP/SR matrix and examples of completed matrix quadrants. Set aside at least 20–30 minutes to complete your matrix and some additional time to answer the self-reflection questions that follow. Although this will not be a formal meditation, it is best to find a quiet and safe space where you can work on this in a mindful and open way. As much as you can, bring a quality of presence, acceptance, and engaged mindful attention to your work with the matrix. After all, you are aiming to inhabit the perspective of an observer, contacting the present moment as you discriminate between valued aims and those behaviors that cause you struggle and suffering. What better quality of mind to bring to such an activity than mindful acceptance, and perhaps even some self-compassion? As you begin, take a few moments to center yourself, practice mindful breathing, and gather your attention.

- First, write your name across the center of the diagram. Then, bring your attention to the first quadrant of the diagram, the bottom right quadrant.
- Now, take a moment and bring to mind what is important to you in your ACT SP/SR work. Bring to mind the problem area that you have been working with throughout this workbook. Consider the following questions:
  - "What is most important to me in this area?"
  - "As I face this problem, what qualities of doing and being do I wish to manifest?"
  - "What do I most value in facing this situation?"
  - "How do I wish to be in my relationships with others around this?"
  - "If I were being the version of myself that I most wish to be, how would I be acting?"

- After you've spent some time with these questions, write your responses in the first quadrant. Write your responses as aspirations to action, often with words ending in *ing*, pointing to how you wish to be. The example of Laura's completed quadrant below illustrates how this process can take shape.

 LAURA'S EXAMPLE: My Values

> **My Values: What qualities of doing, being, and relating matter most to me?**
>
> *Being a skillful, mindful, and compassionate clinician.*
> *Embodying validation, warmth, and strength as a psychotherapist.*
> *Putting my clients' well-being first in our work together.*
> *Supporting my colleagues and receiving support from them.*
> *Helping my clients to live their values out loud.*
> *Helping my clients to find their voice.*
> *Supporting a flow of compassion between myself and my clients that translates into action.*

- Next, bring your attention to the bottom left quadrant, our second quadrant to be addressed. This quadrant asks about those unwanted private experiences that can hook you into cycles of struggle. Sometimes, these thoughts even block or get in the way of your living the values that you just identified. Bring to mind the problem area that you have chosen for this workbook and allow yourself to think of the difficult mental events that are involved in this problem. As much as you can, be open to noticing the worries, ruminations, and self-criticism that might show up concerning this situation. Now, consider the following questions for your SP/SR values:
  - "What unwanted thoughts, feelings, and imaginings can hook me and cause me to struggle with suffering?"
  - "What mental events show up that can get in the way of my moving toward who or what is important to me?"
  - "What are the mental events that I am least willing to feel and that seem to drive my problems in this area?"
- Now, take a moment and fill in your responses in the second quadrant. What thoughts and private events do you notice that are central to your suffering in this area? Laura's example below shows the range of mental experiences that can tie us up in unwanted experience and sometimes direct our attention away from taking action to realize our valued aims.

 LAURA'S EXAMPLE: My Hooks

> **My Hooks: What unwanted thoughts and feelings might get in the way?**
>
> *Anxiety and shame.*
> *Self criticism.*

> Social comparisons.
> Doubting my abilities/knowledge.
> Frustration with "resistant" clients.
> Urges to fix and problem solve.
> Feeling like there is not enough time.
> I am not enough.

- Next, focus in the upper left-hand quadrant, the third quadrant, where you will notice and list patterns of behavior that involve attempts to avoid your "hooks" and unwanted experiences. For this workbook example, choose patterns of avoidance and overcontrol that you use to struggle with your experience of the problem area you have chosen to follow throughout your initial ACT SP/SR journey.

- Here we notice those attempts at EA that typically "backfire" or result in unhealthy patterns or smaller lives. These are the patterns of behavior that sometimes pull us farther from valued action, as we engage in suppressive, avoidant, or addictive ways of being and doing. Now, consider the following questions:

  - "What do I usually do when my mental hooks show up?"
  - "What do I do to get rid of or avoid these hooks?"
  - "What physical changes in body posture or nonverbal behavior might I notice in this area?"
  - "Do I notice any changes in my tone of voice, or pace of speech, when I am more avoidant?"
  - "Are there other visible behaviors I engage in to deal with unwanted mental events?"
  - "What patterns of action do I engage in that serve the function of pushing away unwanted thoughts and feelings?"
  - "What unhelpful, addictive, or avoidant patterns am I engaging in that are failing me, or hurting me?"

- After considering these questions, take a moment to write your responses in the third quadrant of the matrix. You can look at Laura's example below to see some of the ways that she notices herself hooked into avoidant patterns of action.

 LAURA'S EXAMPLE: My Identified Avoidant Patterns of Action

My Identified Avoidant Patterns of Action

> "Rescuing" clients in distress by taking control of the dialogue and colluding in avoidance.
> Trying to fit too much into a session or running overtime in sessions.
> Not asking for help, trying to figure things out alone, overresearching others' problems.

> Getting hooked into "problem-solving mode" rather than staying with a psychological flexible mode.
>
> Sacrificing too much time from other areas of my life or work for clinical work and research—"overworking."
>
> Procrastinating or distracting with social media, TV—"checking out."
>
> Challenging my thoughts and harshly judging myself for having negative thoughts in the first place.
>
> Getting stuck in a cycle of overwork—feeling burned out—and checking out.
>
> Eating takeout food.
>
> "Falling asleep" with the TV on and not getting enough quality sleep at regular times.

- In the final, fourth quadrant, consider what it would look like if you were to move toward these values. Ask yourself:

  - "What would my embodying these values look like?"
  - "What habits and practices can I reliably engage in to serve my valued aims?"
  - "What would it look like if I were engaging in valued behaviors?"
  - "What are some small acts or a personal practice that would begin moving me toward these values?"
  - "What would help me embody these values?"

- Take a few moments and write down your responses in the upper right quadrant. Laura's example below can help as you consider what practices are right for you and your specific valued path through this difficult situation.

 LAURA'S EXAMPLE: My "Toward Moves"

> **My "Toward Moves": My values-focused practices and habits**
>
> Slowing down in sessions and in between sessions.
>
> Mindfully returning to my case conceptualization when I feel rushed.
>
> Speaking to myself from a place of self-compassion, reminding myself that I do know the next right steps.
>
> Noticing when I feel emotionally overextended by an exchange and practicing centering and grounding techniques.
>
> Asking for support/case consultation from colleagues when needed.
>
> Maintaining my sitting meditation practice.
>
> Engaging in restorative leisure activities.
>
> Exercising regularly.
>
> Maintaining good sleep/wake hygiene.
>
> Receiving support from loving and understanding family relationships.

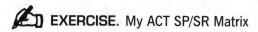 **EXERCISE.** My ACT SP/SR Matrix

My Identified Avoidant Patterns of Action	**My "Toward Moves": My values-focused practices and habits**
My Hooks: What unwanted thoughts and feelings might get in the way?	**My Values: What qualities of doing, being, and relating matter most to me?**

The work we are embarking on together is about creating the conditions where choice becomes available. Together, we are building a life where you create and maintain the choice to move toward who or what is important to you, being the version of yourself you most wish to be, as much as you can. We commit to make this choice, beginning again constantly, even in the presence of obstacles, such as those things you don't want to think or feel. In this way, we realize and manifest psychological flexibility, compassion for ourselves, and transform our lives. Through this process of noticing, making choices, and taking committed action, we have the opportunity to recognize and experience lives of meaning, purpose, and vitality.

Self-Reflective Questions

What was your experience as you engaged in the ACT matrix, working with your individual problem area?

_____

_____

_____

_____

_____

_____

_____

_____

_____

_____

_____

_____

_____

How did you understand our experience of noticing and sorting dimensions of your thoughts and actions into the matrix diagram?

_____

_____

_____

_____

_____

_____

_____

_____

_____

_____

_____

_____

How workable are the strategies in the third quadrant? Have they gotten rid of any of those unwanted inner experiences for good? How are your attempts at avoidance and overcontrol working?

_____

_____

_____

_____

_____

_____

_____

_____

_____

_____

_____

_____

_____

_____

Which life would you choose if you were presented with two options: mostly doing things to move away from what you don't want to feel or think, or mostly doing things to move toward who or what is important to you? What differences would there be in these ways of doing and being?

_____

_____

_____

_____

_____

_____

_____

_____

_____

_____

_____

_____

Did anything in particular stand out or seem important to you in terms of how you can enhance your clinical work? Were there implications for your therapist self that emerged from working with the matrix that might have surprised you?

_____

_____

_____

_____

_____

_____

_____

_____

_____

_____

_____

Were there challenges or areas of difficulty for you in this experience? If so, what were the most challenging dimensions of this practice? What does your experience of this difficulty suggest to you, in terms of your development as a clinician?

_____

_____

_____

_____

_____

_____

_____

_____

_____

_____

_____

_____

_____

How does this work with the matrix change the way you might approach the problem area you are working with, moving forward, in your personal and professional life?

_____

_____

_____

_____

_____

_____

_____

_____

_____

_____

_____

_____

SECTION B

CENTERED

Contacting the Present Moment

Our life is always happening now. Now is the only time you have ever directly experienced. We don't always experience time this way, but it is not a new idea. Throughout human history, many have noted how present-moment experiencing is all we really have and suffering often ensues when we fight this reality or get sucked into thoughts of the past or future. As John Lennon put it in his song "Beautiful Boy (Darling Boy)," "Life is what happens to you while you're busy making other plans." Despite our human abilities to remember, imagine, abstract, change perspectives, and even to think about our thinking, all of these mental experiences are brought forth through cognition—our experience ultimately proceeds from the present. Our direct experiences all unfold here, in this present moment, and "here and now" is the only place/time where/when we can experience ourselves, our world, and our lives. Nonetheless, deliberately holding flexible and focused attention on the present moment can be very challenging. We can get fused and sucked into our thoughts about our experience—we worry about the future, ruminate about the past, and engage in a range of experiential avoidance strategies, all the while moving away from the present, away from our lives. Accordingly, learning to contact and center oneself in present-moment experience helps us return to living our lives and knowing ourselves.

Contacting the present moment in part involves tracking what is happening in the environment right now. We tend to get pulled out of what is happening around us by attending to what our minds are telling us. Try this: Take the book that you are reading right now and hold it against your face. Now, try to read it. We tend to walk around our days in a very similar way, missing what is happening around us while we think about what is happening, has happened, or is going to happen. Just like that book, when our thoughts are focused on the past or future, what is really right in front of us gets blocked. Our private events become a filter through which we experience the world and take it as reality. But what are your thoughts telling you? What is reality? Is your thought about how you aren't working hard enough or is your thought not as "real" as the table in front of you? The music playing from the speakers? Or the book in your hand? Although our thoughts seem very real to us, they are not *us*, and they can pull us away from what is really accessible to us, right now.

When we return our attention and center ourselves in the present moment, several things become available to us. In the ACT model of psychological flexibility, returning to the present moment facilitates defusion, acceptance, and other core psychological flexibility processes. In this way, present-moment awareness is an essential, foundational process in learning and practicing ACT (Hayes et al., 2012). This ability is considered vital for both therapist and client, during ACT sessions and throughout daily life.

The key to maintaining present-moment-focused attention involves the act of returning one's attention back to the present when it has strayed. Rather than training our mind to relentlessly hold one point of focus for an impossible span, we learn to hold our focus on the here and now, and to return this focus to the present whenever it has strayed to responding to imaginal events. This skill is best learned through deliberate practice. This practice can involve deliberate "formal" methods, like seated mindfulness meditation or audio exercises. Examples of the formal practice of contacting the present moment in ACT SP/SR include mindfulness of the breath, the body, the senses, or the present moment itself; other meditation or imagery exercises; and attention training. ACT also involves "informal" practices that help us to deploy present-moment-focused attention while engaging in common tasks. As Golemen and Davidson (2017) suggest in their model of mindfulness, practice in contacting the present moment can at first involve inducing a "state" of mindfulness, and proceed to cultivating a "trait" of mindfulness. In this module, we explore contacting the present moment in ACT, and consider how we might build and maintain a personal present-moment awareness training practice.

Training Contact with the Present Moment in ACT SP/SR

Historically, ACT therapists have been strongly encouraged to have their own mindfulness or present-moment awareness training practice. The reasons for this are due to the experiential nature of mindful awareness and echo the rationale for SP/SR for therapists in general. Thus, ACT SP/SR also emphasizes the importance of regular personalized practice. Much of what we do and teach in ACT is about expanding behavioral repertoires through experiential learning. This requires an understanding of these experiences on multiple levels, including declaratively, procedurally, and experientially.

EXERCISE. Contacting Present-Moment Experience in ACT SP/SR

The following exercise can be used in groups, individually, or in the room with clients. It is a foundational mindfulness exercise that uses the breath as an anchor for the present moment and where you will return to when your mind wanders away from it. You will likely recognize this as a variation of the form of mindful breathing that is widely practiced in Western psychotherapies, and that we explored earlier in this workbook. These experiential exercises are often done in a seated position. You may choose to sit on a straight-back chair with your legs uncrossed, on a meditation cushion, or even on some pillows. It is good to keep your feet on the floor while sitting in a chair. If you are on a cushion, allow your knees to rest on the floor. In this way, you will feel more grounded. For those not using a chair, if you are familiar with the postures involved in seated meditation, you may use such a posture. If these postures are unfamiliar, it is no problem at all—you can just sit in a position that feels supported and comfortable to you. The main aim here is to keep your back in a straight yet relaxed posture. This will allow you to take a deep and full breath and use the full capacity of your diaphragm and lungs. In order to do this, it is a good idea to keep the knees lower than the hips, so that you are less likely to lean or slump forward. This might take a little getting used to, as we aren't always accustomed to sitting with an erect and self-supporting posture, but it is likely to feel quite natural with just a little practice. You might want to imagine a thin invisible thread gently pulling the top of your head toward the ceiling, with your neck relatively free from tension. You can download an audio file of this practice from the book's website (see the box at the end of the table of contents)—alternatively, you can read and memorize the following as guidelines for silent practice.

Our earlier versions of mindfulness of breath and centering practices in this workbook have been very brief. For this version, we ask you to extend your mindfulness of breath practice to 20 minutes. Furthermore, we are leaving longer periods of silence throughout this practice. Notice the effect of remaining in the presence of silence, and extending your experience of the present moment. In your group discussions and self-reflection practices, you might wish to discuss and contrast the experience of sitting for brief periods of time, and sitting for longer periods.

As you begin, allow your eyes to close. Bring your awareness to your feet flat on the floor and then the muscles in your legs. Next, noticing your seat on the chair or cushion, your spine straight and supported, all the way to the top of your head and everything in between. Feel your weight in the chair and notice the volume of space you occupy, here and now.

Bring part of your attention to the sounds around you in the room. As much as you can, notice the space around you through hearing. Now, bring part of your attention to the sounds outside of the room. Finally, bring your attention to the sounds that are farther away, even than that.

On the next inhalation, gently bring your awareness to your breathing, allowing your attention to be with each inhale and each exhale. The breath is always there with us, cycling through us with each inhale and each exhale. There is no need to breathe in any particular way. Simply noticing the experience of breathing. Allowing each breath to flow in its own rhythm. Observe the movement of the breath in the body, taking note of the physical sensations that accompany the flow of breath. It is the nature of our mind to wander and drift away from the breath. When we notice this drift of attention, we may even briefly acknowledge ourselves for having a moment of self-awareness, and gently return our attention to the flow of the breath.

When you are breathing in, knowing you are breathing in.

When you are breathing out, knowing you are breathing out.

Focusing your awareness on the movement of the breath in the abdomen. Observe whatever sensations are present in the abdomen, allowing your attention to collect and gather on the inhalation, and letting go of the awareness of particular sensations as you exhale.

Allow yourself to settle into this awareness, abiding in a state of bare observation of your sensations of breathing, suspending judgment, evaluation, or even description. With your next natural inhale, gently guide your awareness to any other sensations that accompany the breath—perhaps the sensation of cool air in your throat or nostrils as you breathe in or the feeling of warm air as you release and exhale.

When you are breathing in, it is as if you are filling the body with awareness.

When you are breathing out, it is as if you are letting go.

After spending some time observing the breath and you are ready to complete the exercise, with the next available inbreath, expand your awareness to your body. Noticing your feet flat on the floor, the muscles in your legs, your seat on the chair or cushion, your spine straight and supported, all the way to the top of your head and everything in between. When you are ready, you can open your eyes, and bringing this awareness with you into the next moment and those that follow.

Mindfulness and the Human Experience

Paying attention on purpose to the here and now without judgment, evaluation, or resistance is not our default way of being in the world. Our human capacity for symbolic representation and languaging gives rise to our abilities for complex conceptualizations and cognitive processes. All of these unique advantages can have great benefits—in fact, they seem to make mindfulness humanly possible, but can also be the source of great suffering. Our capacity to respond to private events as if they are real can result in reliving past experiences or imagining future ones as if they were occurring right now, all the while, missing out on the moments of our lives as they occur (Wilson & Du Frene, 2009). What is lost in the automatic and distracted nature of our day-to-day functioning are our lives, countless moments, and opportunities to choose our valued ways of being and living.

Troublesome past thoughts tend to be filled with regret, guilt, shame, and depressogenic notions, whereas bothersome future-oriented thoughts lean toward fear, worry, and anxiety. But where is the room for now? Breaking through difficult past and future-oriented thoughts by way of contacting the present moment allows us to create more space for the here and now. Just know that our conceptualized self will show up—on that you can rely. We cannot control what pops into our head—that's the way the mind works. The skill to be practiced here is noticing when distraction arrives, and then using your observer self to bring you back to now.

The present moment is where our ability to act skillfully, flexibly, and make valued choices lives. Right here, in the right now, is where flexibility, self-as-process, and valued living become available to us. By cultivating this centering capacity, the present moment can represent a doorway through which we can return to ourselves as active players in our lives, with meaning and purpose.

Contacting the present moment is a capacity that takes time and practice to build and become more natural. We emphasize this upfront because we hear from clients and trainees frequently that they have difficulty staying in the present moment. If this is true for you, welcome! That's a very human and ubiquitous experience. Recognizing and acknowledging that this is part of the process—and not an exception to it—is key. Noticing when you have lost contact with the now is essential to the ability to return and attend to the present moment. Our next experiential exercise focuses on expanding your awareness to all of your private experiences as they arise in the present moment, followed by your SP/SR reflection questions.

Contacting Thoughts, Feelings, and Sensations in the Present Moment

EXERCISE. "Formal" Practice

Find a place that is quiet and free from distraction. Take a few moments to allow yourself to become comfortable where you're sitting. As you begin this exercise, make any small adjustments to your position and posture that you may need. So that you prepare yourself and your body for this practice, adopt a posture that is secure and grounded.

As you begin, allow your eyes to close. Begin to gently bring part of your attention to the soles of your feet. Next, bring part of your attention to the top of your head. And now, to everything in between. With your next natural inhale, allow your awareness to settle with the sensations of the breath. Breathing in, knowing that you are breathing in, and breathing out, knowing that you are breathing out. Observe the movement of the breath in the body, taking note of the physical sensations that accompany the flow of breath in your body.

It is the nature of our mind to wander and drift away. When we notice this drift of attention, we may even briefly acknowledge ourselves for having a moment of self-awareness, and gently return our attention to the flow of the breath.

With your next natural inhale, allow yourself to expand this awareness to the level of physical sensations that are present throughout your body. If there are feelings of tension, pressure, or discomfort, bring your attention to these as well. As much as you can, bring an attitude of willingness to these experiences. As you breathe in, breathe attention especially into those areas of the body that present you with discomfort, tension, or resistance. Can you make space for these experiences? Bring part of your attention to the feeling of resistance, to the struggle that you are experiencing around these sensations. When meeting each of these sensations, throughout the body, let yourself and your sensations be exactly as you are in this moment.

As you exhale, let go of the attention to physical sensations entirely. With the next available natural inhale, bring your attention to your thoughts and emotions. What thoughts do you notice? What emotions are present? We often find ourselves carried away by our thoughts and feelings. It seems so easy to get caught up in the continual flow of mental images, thoughts, and emotions. In this moment, try to see these thoughts and feelings for what they are. If you find you are getting caught up in them, gently return your awareness back to the sensations of the breath. After staying with this practice for a few minutes, allow your attention to refocus on the objects in your mind itself.

As each new thought or image enters your mind, merely notice and observe it. If you wish, you may want to provide a brief descriptive label to each mental event as it arises and falls away. For instance, you may silently say to yourself, "Worry, I am worrying" or "Memory, that is remembering," when such things occur in your mind. All the while allowing them, accepting them in whatever form they take. See whether you can remain with these mental occurrences, creating room for each as they arrive and noticing them leaving.

From time to time, there are distressing or upsetting mental occurrences. As best you can, simply allow yourself to stay with such experiences, just as you have with other mental events in this practice. As you inhale, allow your awareness to collect in this experience, making space for whatever arises. As you exhale, letting go of this awareness and allowing for whatever the next moment has to offer. Using curiosity and close attention to the ways in which these thoughts or feelings emerge, culminate, and ultimately disappear from awareness. Every individual thought or feeling has a beginning and end, never enduring, never permanent. Allow yourself to be an observer of this continual stream, directing your attention to your mind in action.

With your next available inhale, allow yourself to guide your attention to any other experiences available to you right now. Gently guiding your attention and brining open awareness to whatever you are experiencing. As you exhale for a moment, allow yourself to feel a complete willingness to be exactly who you are, right here and right now.

When you are ready to let go of this exercise, with your next natural inhale, expand your awareness to your feet on the ground. Then to your seat in the chair, to your back feeling straight and supported, and to the top of your head. Now, to everything in between. Returning your attention to the breathing and simply follow the breath. As you are breathing in, knowing that you are breathing in, and as you are breathing out, knowing that you are breathing out. When you are ready, open your eyes and allow yourself to let go of this exercise and resume your day.

EXERCISE. "Informal Practice": Mindful Pleasurable Activity

Take a few moments to engage in an activity that you enjoy. Choose something small—perhaps your first cup of coffee in the morning or practicing an instrument you play, or snuggling with a pet or loved one. Now, go do it, but do it with mindful awareness. As best you can, be open and accepting of all your experience in this activity. Pay attention to what you can perceive with your five senses and how you feel in your body, mind, and heart. Simply observe and note these experiences. Once you are done, complete the following questions:

What did you notice?

What did you perceive with your five senses in those moments?

What did you feel in your body? Describe any physical sensations.

What emotion(s) did you experience?

What thoughts showed up?

What urges and responses arose?

Is there anything that you would like to remember about this experience?

On the next page, we provide a form for you to track your practice in contacting the present moment. During the week that you choose to work through this module, use the form to monitor and explore your personal practice. It is best to begin with the mindfulness of breath practice, and then to add either or both of the additional exercises in this module. After you have completed the week of monitored practice, complete the self-reflection questions that follow.

EXERCISE. Tracking Intentional Practice: Contacting the Present Moment

Day and date	What exercise(s) did you practice? What was the time and place of practice?	Formal or informal practice? (F or I)	What did you notice?
Monday __/__/__			
Tuesday __/__/__			
Wednesday __/__/__			
Thursday __/__/__			
Friday __/__/__			
Saturday __/__/__			
Sunday __/__/__			

⛅ Self-Reflective Questions

What was your experience as you engaged in the mindful breathing exercise? What observations were most vivid to you in the moment?

_____

_____

_____

_____

_____

_____

_____

_____

_____

_____

_____

_____

What did you notice as you engaged in the contacting your experience in the present moment exercise? What observations were most vivid to you in this practice?

_____

_____

_____

_____

_____

_____

_____

_____

_____

_____

_____

_____

_____

What was different in these experiences from your everyday awareness and attention?

_____

_____

_____

_____

_____

_____

_____

_____

_____

_____

_____

_____

Was there anything in these experiences you would like to remember? What does this experience, and what you will carry forward, tell you about yourself as a clinician?

_____

_____

_____

_____

_____

_____

_____

_____

_____

_____

_____

_____

How do you plan to practice contacting the present-moment practices going forward? How can you bring greater contact with the present moment forward in your clinical work?

_____

_____

_____

_____

_____

_____

_____

_____

_____

_____

_____

Self-as-Context

A long with the other core psychological flexibility processes, in ACT SP/SR we focus on developing our "self-as-context." As we have discussed, this term points to an "observing self" that is experienced as a consistent "I–here–nowness" of our being, across time and place. This observer perspective contains all of our experience, and is distinct from our "self-story." We train our ability to access and inhabit our self-as-context mode of being through the use of a range of techniques, including metaphors, meditations, and other perspective-taking exercises. In this module and the next, we work with a deepening experience of self-as-context. We also practice differentiating between our narrative of *self-as-content* and our experience of *self-as-context*.

Self-as-Content: The Conceptualized Self

Throughout history, we humans have struggled with the question "Who am I?" That struggle proceeds over the course of one human life, just as it has proceeded over the course of the evolution of our species.

From a very young age, we learn to use words and cognitions to categorize and evaluate our world and our experience, and over time, our self. We build an inner symbolic representation of who we are, relative to others, to the future and to the world. As we have seen, at the root of this process is our ability to derive relations among stimuli, to use internal language, and to judge and define our experience. This human tendency leads us to constantly assess and judge the meaning of our experiences, "good" versus "bad," or "right" versus "wrong." This conceptualizing continues throughout our lives, is part of what makes us human, and allows us to know ourselves. When this process is focused on our sense of self, we can find ourselves with rigid self-concepts or labels, such as "productive," "imposter," or "bad parent." It follows that we all learn to use a variety of evaluations and descriptions to define ourselves—some we like, some we do not. How we learn to respond to our sense of self can either broaden or narrow our behavior and often our lives, depending on our learning history.

Our narrative experience of self can feel so ubiquitous, foundational, and "real" that most of us often mistake our self-concept for an absolute truth about who we are and what life is all about. Funnily enough, our self-experience is just another construct of the mind, and we can learn to relate to this sense of self in radically different ways, with powerful results.

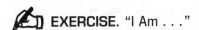 **EXERCISE.** "I Am . . ."

Consider your sense of "self" for a moment and complete the following sentence as quickly as you can, trying not to give it much thought:

"I am _____."

Let's consider a number of questions about your response.

- What came to mind when you were asked to complete the sentence?
- Did you describe a conceptualization of yourself? *(Perhaps you described some part of your narrative history or origin. Maybe you noted some dimension of your identity. For example, you might have written "I am from the south of England," or you might have stated "I am a doctoral student.")*
- Is the self-concept that you wrote above new or old?
- Does the answer represent all of who you are?
- What are the other ways you could have completed this sentence?
- What thoughts about this sentence do you have?
- What emotions or sensations are you feeling as you read these words?
- As you notice your responses to these questions, here and now, consider the following question: *Who is it that is noticing all of this?*

Our behavior of constructing a conceptualized experience of a separate self through describing and evaluating our "selves" is called our "narrative self," or self-as-content in ACT. Our experience of our self-as-content can be similar to looking at the "table of contents" of our life's story. We designate labels for ourselves and our experiences, and somehow pull together a narrative structure that helps us make sense of our experience and our actions. In ACT, self-as-content is often referred to as the "story" that our mind creates about who we are and what we experience.

When we become too fixed or reliant on these conceptualizations, ineffective, inflexible, and sometimes harmful behavior can result. We have evolved to seek adherence to our self-imposed verbal rules. Thus, our self-identities can circumscribe us, condition our behaviors, and limit our experiences. We come to believe that our experiences and our responses to them define us and that our destiny relies on them. Thus, we find ourselves playing out complex versions of our mind's own self-fulfilling prophecy.

Excessively defining ourselves by our self-concepts can have a deleterious effect on our psychological flexibility.

When we become overly fused with our conceptualization of self, our lives can become smaller and we tend to suffer as a result. It's no wonder that self-esteem has been one of the most researched topics in psychology. Indeed, when we overidentify or fuse with a negative or unhelpful conceptualized self, realizing our deepest values in life can feel impossible.

Research has demonstrated that chronic shame and self-criticism are transdiagnostic factors in psychotherapy that contribute to a great deal of human suffering, and that can confound treatment effectiveness (Gilbert, 2011). When we are confronted by the perceived impact of limiting or destructive self-concepts, we might understandably believe that we should work to directly change our negative thoughts about ourselves, work to increase our "self-esteem," or somehow become a "better person."

ACT offers freedom from the tyranny of fusion with our conceptualized self through flexible perspective taking. In ACT, we intentionally access an experience of *self-as-context* to broaden the experience of the self and broaden the possibilities of our experience and action.

In ACT, we find an alternative to strategies that are based primarily on challenging or "restructuring" our *self-as-content* story. Rather than focusing our mental training on correcting, disputing, or modifying our self-conceptualizations, in ACT, we practice shifting our perspective from that of the individual protagonist in a self-story to that of an "observing self" (Deikman, 1982; Harris, 2009). We practice noticing and holding our self-stories lightly rather than situating our experience within a reified sense of self in compliance with our personal narratives. In a sense, ACT is about learning new ways to respond to our sense of self. Our focus is not on how "negative" or "positive" our self-conceptualizations are but instead on *changing our relationship* to our self-stories and *loosening the grip they have on us*.

✍ EXERCISE. The Ocean of Being

The meditation below is designed to help us contact our experience of self-as-context by using mindfulness, rhythmic breathing, and imagery. As with all of our mediations and experiential exercises in this workbook, it is best to practice in a safe and quiet environment where you will be undisturbed for approximately 15 minutes. This practice can be used as an introduction to the experience of inhabiting your observing self, and it can also be used as a daily practice. When used daily, we are deliberately using imagery to cultivate our experience of what is called the "ground of being" in Tibetan Vajrayana Dzogchen Buddhist practice (Dalai Lama, 2004). Indeed, the deeply meditative imagery practice below has much in common with meditations in such lineages. However, for our experiential exercise, we don't need any advanced meditation training, nor do we need to hold any belief system. We are simply using our imagination to contact an experience of self that allows us to hold all of our experience in bare attention, moment by moment, from the perspective of our self-as-context. You can download an audio version of this practice from the book's website (see the box at the end of the table of contents). Alternatively, you can read and record the instructions below, or eventually internalize and memorize the following as guidelines for your own, ongoing silent practice.

Begin by closing your eyes and allowing yourself a long and relaxing exhalation. As you exhale, imagine that you are releasing any needless tension that you might be clinging to in this moment. As you breathe in, notice any places that your body might be tensing up, preparing you for some action, or even providing extra rigidity and support. With your next, long exhalation, release the tension that you have just noticed.

As you continue with a slow, mindful pace of breath, allow yourself to adjust your position in your chair or meditation cushion so that you feel stabilized and grounded. As much as you can, adopt a dignified and solid posture, embodying the qualities of dignity, centeredness, and authority within yourself. It is as if there is an invisible thread that gently pulls your head and spine into alignment, supporting you as it disappears into the clouds far above.

With our next inhale, we bring part of our attention to the soles of our feet. Exhaling, we bring part of our attention to the top of the head. Continuing with our mindful breathing, we fill our body with an awareness of everything in between. Now, bring awareness to the sounds that you hear in the room, the sounds just outside of the room, and the sounds that are farther away, even than that.

With the next inbreath, it is as if we are breathing attention into the body, filling the body with the presence of life. With the next outbreath, it is as if we are letting go. Follow your breath in this way, gathering your attention, and letting it go, with each cycle of your breath.

Breathing in, allowing yourself to feel awake, alert, and alive. Breathing in, allowing yourself to feel centered and grounded. Adopting as open and accepting an awareness as you can, with every moment. As we do, when thoughts arise, we make space for whatever has arisen. Noticing the thought, image, or emotion, and gently bringing your attention back to the flow of your breathing with the next natural inbreath.

As you follow the breath, allow each outbreath to lengthen, extending the rhythm of your breath and slowing down. We are slowing the body, and slowing the mind. Gradually, we approach a rhythm of just a few breaths per minute. Allow your breath to breathe itself in this way, and to find its own focused and centered rhythm.

Remain with the silence and your breath, holding yourself in kindness and resting in the breath for the next few minutes.

When you are ready, begin to turn the focus of your mindful awareness to the thoughts themselves. Noticing how each mental event proceeds before the ever-present witness that is your observing self. You, as the observer, can watch the arising of each thought. Notice how the thought begins. In this moment, watching how the thought proceeds and how it changes. Observing how the thought flows and begins to complete itself. In this very moment, observe how the thought ends. Notice the space between one thought and the arising of the next thought. Resting in this moment, observe the flow of these thoughts, as much as you can.

Taking some time to simply remain in the presence of your mental events, you are awake, alert, and alive. Begin to allow an image to form in your mind. This image is of yourself standing on a beach.

The beach is inviting, beautiful, and calm. It is early in the morning, you are alone, and the sunlight is warm, while the breeze is cooling. This may be a beach you are creating from memory, or a beach that your mind is creating for you from pure imagination. You can see the sunlight flickering across the surface of the water like dancing diamonds. You can feel the sand beneath your feet. Breathing in, knowing that you are breathing in. Breathing out, knowing that you are breathing out.

Imagine that each of your thoughts is represented by one of the waves that gently rolls in from the ocean. Each wave is one of your thoughts. Each thought is one of the waves. Notice how the wave begins, seemingly rolling out from the horizon.

In this moment, watching how the wave proceeds and how it flows and changes in shape and size. Observing how each wave of thought rolls forward and begins to complete itself. In this very moment, observe how the wave graces the shore. Notice how some thought waves come to an end softly, resolving into the beach, watching as some waves of thought crash onto the shore. Notice the space between one wave of thought and the arising of the next wave. Resting in this moment, observe the flow of these thought waves, as much as you can. As you watch the waves, you are the observer, you are not the waves themselves, but they unfold before you, again and again, and always in this present moment. This one moment is every moment, and it is the only moment. This moment.

Now, imagine that you are no longer watching the waves from the shore, but that you have become the ocean itself. Allow yourself to expand, and to become this ocean. Keeping part of our attention in our breath, breathing in and knowing we are breathing in, and breathing out and knowing we are breathing out, we can feel ourselves being the ocean. Just as the ocean, we are impossibly deep and wide. We can feel the spaciousness and interiority of our being. Allow yourself to rest in silence for a few moments and to feel this space within.

You are the ocean, here and now.

Just as the ocean has waves, but is far more than any one wave, you have mental events—thoughts, images, memories, and sensations. Just as waves move through the ocean, and move as the ocean, your mental events move through you and in you. You are so much more than any one thought. You are so much more than any one story. In this moment, resting in the breath and holding ourselves in kindness, we can allow the flow of our waves of experience to move through us, as we are the deep and wide ocean.

Rest in silence and observe the waves moving through you. Notice this oceanic self, which is strong, flowing, and able to make space for all things in all directions. Rest in this way of being, in this ocean of being, for as long as you wish.

Taking some time outside of clock time, bringing our attention to this natural inbreath, we are beginning to let go of the imagery. With each breath, our attention is more fully focused on the here and now experience of breathing itself.

In this moment, allowing yourself some gratitude for practicing something new and for expanding your experience, and beginning to form an intention to let go of this practice altogether.

With our next inhale, we bring part of our attention to the soles of our feet. Exhaling, we bring part of our attention to the top of our head. Continuing with our mindful breathing, we fill our body with an awareness of everything in between. Now, bring awareness to the sounds that you hear in the room, the sounds just outside of the room, and the sounds that are farther away, even than that.

When you are ready, open your eyes, return your attention to the room around you, stretch if you feel like it, and prepare to let this practice go and to return to the flow of your day.

🗨 *Self-Reflective Questions*

What was your experience of self-as-context during the reading and experiential practices found in this module?

_____

_____

_____

_____

_____

_____

_____

_____

_____

_____

_____

How do you understand your experience of self-as-context?

_____

_____

_____

_____

_____

_____

_____

_____

_____

_____

_____

_____

_____

In what ways does viewing our mental events from the perspective of self-as-context affect us? How does this capacity show up in your clinical practice and in the psychotherapy relationship?

_____

_____

_____

_____

_____

_____

_____

_____

_____

_____

_____

How might you bring a self-as-context perspective to bear on the problem area that you have chosen to work with in this workbook? How might this enhance your clinical work?

_____

_____

_____

_____

_____

_____

_____

_____

_____

_____

_____

_____

How do you understand the relationship between viewing your present-moment experience from the perspective of the observer and your ability to live your values more fully as you face the challenging problem that you have been working with throughout our ACT SP/SR program? In your personal life? In your professional life?

_____

_____

_____

_____

_____

_____

_____

_____

_____

_____

_____

MODULE 7

Flexible Perspective Taking

Our work with self-as-context is grounded in the contextual science of perspective taking (Foody, Barnes-Holmes, & Barnes-Holmes, 2012; Hayes et al., 2012). Earlier perspective-taking techniques in ACT were primarily centered on using our capacity for intentionally shifting perspective to access the "observing self," as we have explored in the previous module. However, over the last two decades, ACT and CBS technologies have expanded and developed to use a range of "flexible perspective-taking" techniques that can enhance our psychological flexibility (McHugh, Stewart, & Hooper, 2012; Yadavaia, Hayes, & Vilardaga, 2014; Yu, Norton, & McCracken, 2017).

Drawing upon the corpus of RFT research and translating the science to user-friendly terms, Harris has described the expansive importance of flexible perspective taking as follows:

> The less common meaning of self-as-context is "flexible perspective-taking." When used with this meaning, self-as-context refers to any and all types of flexible perspective-taking; which are all classed as "deictic framing" in relational frame theory. Flexible perspective-taking underlies defusion, acceptance, contacting the present moment, self-awareness, empathy, compassion, theory of mind, and mental projection into the future or past. (*www.actmindfully.com.au/upimages/Making_Self-As-Context_Relevant,_Clear_and_Practical.pdf*)

In RFT, "deictic framing" refers to a pattern of relating stimuli in terms of the perspective of the experiencer (McHugh et al., 2012). The most common frames we discuss in terms of deictic framing are the experiences of *I and you,* of *here and there,* and of *then and now.* As individuals cultivate greater flexibility and fluency in their ability to take perspective through deictic framing, they may develop greater psychological flexibility and mental agility. Accordingly, the ACT community has been honing the use of flexible perspective taking through psychotherapy techniques that translate well to our ACT SP/SR work.

Beyond our scientific grounding in RFT, it is worth noting that many psychotherapy approaches share perspective taking as a means to shed a different light on our day-to-day experiences as humans. This is often present in therapists' encouraging a more longitudinal view of our human experience, as opposed to our being caught up with the day-to-day minutiae of our lived experience. For example, patients with depression tend to notice that their thoughts are often littered with regrets and recriminations regarding events in their life where they are locked into a perspective that they should have behaved "better" or done a "better" job. Simply shifting perspective to how they might view a beloved friend who faced the same challenges can go a long way to getting unhooked from fusion with this perspective. Similarly, people who struggle with anxiety often notice that their thoughts are predominantly guided by a "What if?" filter whereby the reflections are taken up with worry about how their actions might impinge on the well-being of others or themselves. Imagining these worries from different points in time, place, and person can loosen the grip of the worries on our actions and states of being.

As therapists, we can perhaps relate to these human struggles. Given the compassionate motivation of humans who are drawn toward caring for others, we are driven toward perhaps wanting to "make a difference" or wishing to be the person who does not "let others down."

Of course, one can notice a direct link to our values—that within the preceding statement. We can notice a wish to alleviate suffering, or at least to not knowingly cause harm to ourselves or others. Nonetheless, living the struggle that we often experience as humans, we often fail and we often suffer. Our experience can be guided by what is important to us, and yet the narrow focus of a self-as-content-driven perspective can drive us into self-blame, as we minimize the weight and influence of the context of our human experience.

As CFT founder Paul Gilbert (2010) has often described, we don't get to choose how our minds operate; our mental functioning is an evolutionary "gift" to us. Also, we don't tend to choose our learned history. For example, if we have been abducted from our safe learning environments as children and thrust into abusive and criminalized environments, it is likely that we would adapt to our experience and act and behave in a way that is far divorced from the life that we would wish for ourselves. It can be useful to adopt a perspective where we realize how much in life that drives our suffering is not of our choosing, and is not our fault. This simple act of perspective taking—holding the big picture of our human condition and recognizing how much is just not our fault—can go a long way. We begin where we are. We move forward by coming from. Where we find ourselves we do the best that we can. It is often noticed, for example, that as humans we tend to be more forgiving of others' human frailties and yet are our own worst critics in viewing our own transgressions of a similar nature. May we be able to stand back from our self-blame and from fusion with self-evaluative and condemning self-statements, so that we might be better able to mindfully embody and realize our valued aims.

This module therefore is *less* concerned with searching for different perspectives from *others'* lived experience, which indicates that wisdom is found elsewhere. We are more interested in flexing and transforming our perspective itself, and in casting a compassionate light on our own lived human experience. Perhaps we might even recognize that we do the best that we can in the place in which we find ourselves much of the time.

So, while it may be likely that in terms of perspective taking we tend to think initially of others' wisdom, the heart of this module is considering how we can bring our own compassion and wisdom to our own lived human experience in the various contexts that we have found ourselves. You can download an audio version of this practice from the book's website (see the box at the end of the table of contents), or record yourself reading the instructions and play them back.

✍️ EXERCISE. Time Travel

Take a moment and bring to mind a time when you have been struggling with thoughts and feelings related to the problem area you have been working on. You might wish to take a couple of minutes to practice mindful breathing and to center and focus. Close your eyes and allow an image of the situation to form in your mind. As much as you can, bring to mind this recent time, and imagine that you are there now. Imagine the details of the place and the sensory experiences. What was going through your mind when you were the you who was there and then, rather than the you who is here and now? Remember who you were with, what you were doing, and what was on your mind.

Next, shift your perspective on the situation and the events so that you can see your past self, as though you were an invisible visitor in the room. Rather than seeing the situation by looking out through the eyes of your past self, imagine that you are a silent observer of the situation. See whether you can look at this person who is suffering with the same kindness, understanding, and empathy that you would have for a very good friend. When you look into the eyes of your past self, see the concern, the distress, and the difficult experience that this human is going through and extend your care and acceptance toward them.

Let's imagine that you could travel in time to transport back to the moment of distress and suffering that you are imagining. This is a moment that is in the past. While you were distressed and entangled with your thoughts at that time, you are now in a place that feels safer, practicing mindfulness. You have the benefit of a different perspective and the shift in understanding that can come with hindsight. If you could take that time machine back to that moment, and the you who is here and now could contact the you who was there and then, what might this version of you say to your past self? How might your present moment self-engage with your past self in a useful way? Perhaps more importantly, what would your past self say to this future self, who has come out of nowhere with some helpful words? Would the suggestions be well received? If your past self would resist the help of the you who is here and now, how might you try to connect and reach that past self with empowering and productive new ways of approaching the situation?

Sit with this exercise for some time and when you are ready, open your eyes and answer the questions below. We also provide an example of how one of us (Dennis) completed this exercise.

EXERCISE. My Time Travel Worksheet

In what situation did you imagine your past self? What was happening? Who was there?	
What thoughts were going through your mind in this situation?	
What emotions did your past self feel in this situation?	
If the present "you"—the "you" who is here and now—could travel back in time to say something useful and encouraging to your past self—the "you" who was there and then—what would that be?	
If your past self could hear these words and feel your compassion and engagement, how might your past self respond to your message?	
If your past self was too entangled in your experience to hear your message, or strongly resisted your communication, what would you say to aim to help?	

EXAMPLE: Dennis's Time Travel Worksheet

In what situation did you imagine your past self? What was happening? Who was there?	My past self was in my car, driving to spend time with my brother, his wife, and their children on a Saturday afternoon. It was a beautiful summer day and we were planning on relaxing beside their swimming pool and barbecuing.
What thoughts were going through your mind in this situation?	"I have really screwed up now. I don't have enough time to complete my writing projects at home, or to attend to my email, and I should be taking care of that this afternoon, not lounging around. But if I don't make time for the people I love, I'm not being fair to them, and I'm not really living. I just hate myself right now. Why can't I manage my responsibilities like a normal person?"
What emotions did your past self feel in this situation?	My past self was feeling a lot of self-directed anger and despair.
If the present "you"—the "you" who is here and now—could travel back in time to say something useful and encouraging to your past self—the "you" who was there and then—what would that be?	"Your writing, your clients, and your work as an ACT therapist really mean a lot to you. So does your family. It is really tough to manage these competing demands and valued aims. You aren't alone, my friend. It is tough for a lot of us. I know you have managed these responsibilities well in the past, and are capable of it now. It is all right for you to practice self-compassion and take some time with family, and then return to your work. Hold the anxiety as lightly as you can, and aim to show up fully for the people you love."
If your past self could hear these words and feel your compassion and engagement, how might your past self respond to your message?	"I know that what you are saying makes sense, but I am just so angry with myself. I can't stand to be stuck on this treadmill where I never really feel free to show up for what I am doing, because there is a mountain of other stuff that needs attention. Thanks for trying to help, but I just want to scream."
If your past self was too entangled in your experience to hear your message, or strongly resisted your communication, what would you say to aim to help?	"Hey man, of course you want to scream! I will scream with you if it helps! Nothing you are feeling is bad in itself, and it is OK to feel it. Let's just feel this fully together. Let's pull over for 3 minutes of mindful acceptance of just how stressful it is to want to be in two places at once, brother! You have committed a lot of yourself to making a difference in the world, from being a loving uncle to being the best trainer and therapist you can be. What would you have to give up caring about in order to not have this stress you out? In your pain you find your values, and in your values you find your pain! Now, let's go swimming with the kids and spend some time in the sun. I've got your back."

✎ EXERCISE. Taking the Perspective of My Most Difficult Client

Bring to mind your most challenging client. Ideally, you are still working with this client, but considering a former client can also be beneficial. Indicate below what makes this person difficult:

☐ They don't seem invested in their therapy.

☐ Their value system differs from yours.

☐ They elicit feelings of incompetence or insecurity.

☐ They have a conflictual interpersonal style.

☐ Their behavior seems destructive and incomprehensible.

☐ Other (list): _____

Even though there may be many factors that make this client a challenge for you, we'd like you to zero in even further by identifying the *most* challenging factor. If you are unable to do this because you find several features equally difficult, take notice of this difficulty and then select a single concern. Once identified, allow yourself to consider, as fully as you can, a recent time when you experienced this difficulty with your client. Allow all of the thoughts, feelings, sensations, and so forth to become fully salient. Take note of what it's like for you to have this experience.

Once this experience is fully present, we'd like you to consider a number of different perspectives. First, try to get inside your client's skin a bit and notice whether you can see the world from their eyes during this recent experience you identified. What might they be thinking? Can you think these thoughts as if you were them? What are they feeling? Can you feel these feelings as you observe the circumstance from their perspective? Can you experience, even if only briefly, their struggle in that moment? Even though their behavior might be ineffective or even destructive, is there another side to their behavior? Could it also make sense and be functional in some ways?

Now, consider where your client might have learned this behavior. Perhaps you know enough about their history to reasonably speculate about this. Maybe it was learned during their younger years. If so, see whether you are able to view the world from their eyes during this period of their life. What were they doing, thinking, and feeling then? Examine this from two perspectives: (1) the client's perspective as a child and (2) your perspective of them then from your current vantage point. Is it possible for you to consider how you might have developed the same behavioral pattern had you experienced the exact same learning history?

Make note what this exercise was like for you and what impact it had, if any, on your struggle with your experience of this client.

Self-Reflective Questions

What was your experience as you engaged in the time travel exercise in flexible perspective taking? What observations were most vivid to you in the moment? What did you learn?

_____

_____

_____

_____

_____

_____

_____

_____

_____

_____

_____

Did you experience a sense of self that was larger than your day-to-day experiences? As best you can do, how would you describe that experience?

_____

_____

_____

_____

_____

_____

_____

_____

_____

_____

_____

_____

What do you make of this experience and what does this tell you about your lived experience as a person? What does this tell you about your experience as an ACT therapist?

_____

_____

_____

_____

_____

_____

_____

_____

_____

_____

_____

How might this experience be helpful in your day-to-day living and clinical practice?

_____

_____

_____

_____

_____

_____

_____

_____

_____

_____

_____

_____

_____

How might flexible perspective taking impact your practice of psychotherapy, generally speaking? When considering your most difficult client, how could perspective taking improve the quality of your care? Would it be useful to develop a regular perspective-taking practice?

_____

_____

_____

_____

_____

_____

_____

_____

_____

_____

_____

SECTION C

OPEN

MODULE 8

Defusion

Defusion represents one of the core processes of being "open" and psychologically flexible in ACT SP/SR. As we have seen, defusion involves undermining the "literality" with which we experience our cognitive representations (Hayes et al., 1999). In simpler terms, this means that we learn how to respond to cognitions as thoughts, in and of themselves, rather than responding to thoughts as though they were actual events taking place in the outside world. Intentionally responding to our thoughts with defusion, as opposed to being "fused with" a thought, has been characterized as "having a thought versus buying a thought" (Hayes, 2005, p. 71). So, when we practice defusion we aim to be better able to respond to thoughts and verbal representations of reality without being excessively controlled by such mental events.

In a sense, defusion practice is not a new approach to thinking. For thousands of years, meditative practices have taught people how to take a step back from their thinking and observe the flow of mental events as the actions of their mind, rather than as reality (Tirch et al., 2015). CBT therapists have long taught clients to "decenter" from their thinking and to examine and analyze their thoughts for their utility and validity, rather than simply believing everything they think (Beck, 2011). Perhaps what distinguishes defusion as a process is the precision and clarity of the focus of defusion exercises. When we practice defusion, we aren't really concerned about whether our thoughts are true or untrue, or even whether they are functional or dysfunctional. We also aren't necessarily aiming to penetrate the illusions of the mental world as a part of realizing the ultimate nature of reality and becoming enlightened (though this is permitted). Defusion seeks to help us to get out from under the excessive influence of our thoughts and mental events so that we can have greater freedom to choose our actions and behaviors in the service of realizing our valued aims. It is that simple and direct.

According to the Greek philosopher Epictetus, "Men are disturbed not by things, but by the view which they take of them" (in Ellis, 1979). Throughout our lives, we experience thoughts and feelings that are at times extremely uncomfortable and certainly unwanted. This is not something within our control but part of the human experience.

Whether this private content determines how we choose to act in our lives is a different matter, and defusion processes within an ACT model seek to address this issue. To this end, the process of cognitive defusion refers to an ongoing process of mindfully noticing our internal verbal world, and deliberately choosing to move toward realizing our values, even when unhelpful thoughts are discouraging or seemingly blocking such actions. This approach to life undermines the idea that "in order to live better, I have to feel better." Some would say that defusion and acceptance are aimed at helping us to get better at feeling, rather than helping us to "feel better" (Harris, 2006; Luoma, Hayes, & Walser, 2007).

What Is Fusion?

In more general usage, the term *fusion* represents a merging or mingling of two or more things to become one thing, such as the fusion of resin and glass fiber to produce fiberglass. Naturally, when we talk about the fusion of psychological experiences, it becomes trickier than describing a blending of observable physical substances. For example, let's imagine that a woman has learned to brutally criticize herself. When she was young, her mother would consistently berate her about being lazy and would yell at her about how important it was to succeed. Spurred on by her fears, the woman studied very hard and achieved academic excellence. Over time, she has come to deeply believe that she is lazy and prone to failure, and that she needs to listen to her inner critic or she will fail. Now, let's imagine that this woman has risen very high in her career, and is the CEO of an international firm. She is ceaselessly hardworking and good-natured in her work. She is highly paid, and also has a loving family and a mostly healthy lifestyle. By all accounts, this woman is successful. Nevertheless, her mind still tells her "You are lazy, and you are ruining your life." When these thoughts arrive, they take hold as if they were an absolute reality. The woman can find herself anxious and depressed, inactive in the face of feelings of worthlessness. More often though, these thoughts drive a kind of "workaholism" where she just can't stop throwing herself into her work, leading to some exhaustion and burnout. The woman is "fused" with her self-criticism, and this can take charge of her life.

In this way, we can become fused is the experience of being "hooked," rather like Velcro, on aspects of our private experience, and more so with the evaluations of them.

Moving from Fusion to Defusion: "Diving In"

What are you fused with? Most of us can identify a very familiar struggle. Perhaps you are stuck ruminating on concerns about work, your love life, family, or self-judgments. The mental events that can come to dominate our lives can have universal themes, while they remain distinctively our own. For the following exercise, the practice of "diving in," we ask you to consider a familiar mental struggle, particularly one that you notice you spend a lot of time with. It would be helpful, for our ACT SP/SR purposes, if this struggle related to the problem you have chosen to focus on while using this workbook. Once you have settled on a particular area of fusion and struggle, formulate a sentence or two that you are very "fused" with. From a centered and mindful place, you will repeatedly ask yourself a question. The question is almost like a mantra, in that it repeatedly brings us into contact with an experience and holds our attention closely to a concept. You will ask yourself "What does my thought say about me?" With each iteration, you will allow yourself to settle in further to the experience of the thought with which you are fused. You will observe the influence that this thought has upon you, and will look more deeply at how this thought exerts an influence upon you.

Similar to practices in "extending" or "vertical descent" (Leahy, 2017), we are looking at the deeper implications of automatic thoughts and cognitive rules. However, unlike older variations of CBT, we are not looking for a structural "core belief" that we wish to change. We are using our observing capacity to notice the function of our thoughts. We are looking at how fusion with a thought has allowed us to surrender some of the quality of our lives to a verbal process. This can open the door to a newer, deeper freedom.

MY FAMILIAR STRUGGLE IS:

In order to help you to frame your struggle, we offer an example of Martin's diving-in log. In Martin's example, he has been struggling with parenting issues and, in particular, has been finding it difficult to manage or to control his feelings about being angry with his daughter.

EXAMPLE: Martin's Diving-In Log

MY FAMILIAR STRUGGLE IS:
I worry about getting frustrated with my teenage daughter. When I think about this, I experience angry feelings that I don't like.

Familiar struggle	Worrying about getting frustrated with my teenage daughter and noticing angry feelings that I don't like.
What does this say about you?	Well, I should be able to control my feelings, and I certainly should not be getting annoyed with my daughter as often as I experience.
And what does this say about you?	I feel weak and helpless, and I worry that I'm pushing her further and further away from me.
And what does this say about you?	I am not doing my job properly and I am not setting a very good example to my daughter.
And what does this say about you?	I'm just not being the parent that I want to be. It upsets me that I just can't get this right.
And what does this say about you?	I'm a failure as a parent and I'm a failure as a person.
And how old is this? For how long have you thought in this way?	Ever since I first became a parent, and before that, I felt like a failure in other ways, for a very long time.

Looking at Martin's example there are various aspects that demonstrate fusion in action from a contextual behavioral perspective. "Well, I should be able to control my feelings" is an important statement. Within personal evaluations, "should" is often indicative of personal rules and certainly suggestive of something being held rigidly (Ellis & Robb, 1994). In Martin's case, the concept is that "feelings should be controlled." Martin exhibits fusion with this rule.

This points to an unworkable solution. If Martin believes that controlling feelings of annoyance means that he will experience less annoyance, there is an abundance of research that indicates that moves to control or suppress unwanted thoughts and feelings can lead to a perceived increase of those same emotions and thoughts rather than a reduction (Wegner & Gold, 1995; Wegner, Schneider, Knutson, & McMahon, 1991; Wenzlaff & Wegner, 2000).

Also, feelings do not come complete with an off/on switch (Bach & Moran, 2008), and while it is understandable that humans might wish to be able to regulate emotions in this way, this is not our experience. For example, imagine that somebody offered you $1 million to fall in love with the next person you see—not simply acting in a loving way or with loving words but actually falling head over heels in love. Do you think that is possible? Can we just choose how we feel? "In our heart," we know this is not the case.

Martin indicates how significant the urge to control feelings is: "I'm just not being the parent that I want to be," "I worry that I am pushing her further and further away," and "I'm a failure as a parent and I'm a failure as a person."

This is important for a number of reasons. First, it clearly demonstrates fusion with self-as-content. Like all people, Martin has countless facets, emotions, experiences, memories, and behaviors, yet he is so caught up with these unwanted feelings that he is unable to perceive the distinction between himself and those feelings—that is, "I experience angry feelings that I don't like." Second, Martin is defining himself as a parent and indeed as a person based on his thoughts and feelings. In other words, "I am a bad parent," and "I am a bad person."

In addition, Martin demonstrates how private events can be perceived to be toxic—his experience of annoyance is evaluated as leading to pushing his daughter away and not being the parent that he wants to be. This also shows fusion with an imagined past or future—clearly, Martin is worrying that if the rule to control his feelings is not followed, then his relationship with his daughter will be in jeopardy. While not explicit in the above exercise, Martin ultimately stating "I'm a failure as a person" is likely to relate to previous evaluations.

Stepping back from the immersion control these thoughts exert on our behaviors is an act of defusion, in and of itself. From this stance, we can approach the question of how familiar the individual is with this stream of thoughts. For how long has a person's life been dominated by these mental events?

"How Old Is This?"

When you have completed the practice below, before answering the last question, refer to your evaluation of "What does this say about me?" and then ask yourself the final question: "And how old is this? For how long have you thought in this way?" It is likely that such a personal evaluation is very familiar and very old. For some of us, our answer might look something like "This has been with me since I can remember. At least since childhood. I have never felt good enough and I worry that I will never get it right."

There is one more significant aspect of the sticky processes of fusion to consider. Let us return to the statements in Martin's example: "I'm just not being the parent that I want to be" and "I'm a failure as a parent." What is often found in the human experience is that which we most struggle with is somehow tied up or fundamentally connected to what matters most to us as humans—our personal values. We explore this further in the modules regarding values.

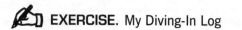 **EXERCISE.** My Diving-In Log

Familiar struggle	
What does this say about you?	
And what does this say about you?	
And what does this say about you?	
And what does this say about you?	
And what does this say about you?	
And how old is this? For how long have you thought in this way?	

Now, let's move on to another form of looking at defusion through a mindfulness practice aimed at finding the separation between you and your thoughts. There is a difference between the thinker and the thoughts. We are pulled to believe we are one and the same, but indeed, that's an illusion. The following exercise assists you in understanding how that is so.

✍️ EXERCISE. Externalizing the Thought

This exercise is designed to demonstrate the difference between who we are as a person and our thoughts as a procession of mental events. This practice involves externalizing and looking at your thoughts using various mental faculties, including visual and imaginal methods. The practice also asks you to be creative and present minded. These are all ways to heighten the experience of defusion, and ways to put space between you and your thoughts, without having to avoid them. Creativity and present-moment awareness are part of the experience of stepping back from the thoughts instead of a way to avoid or replace them. You can download an audio version of this practice from the book's website (see the box at the end of the table of contents), or alternatively, you can read and memorize the following as guidelines for silent practice.

If you are comfortable doing so, close your eyes. If not, fix your gaze on a spot in the room. Follow your breath, in and out, practicing your contact with the present moment, as you have learned. Slow your breath and notice your chest rising and falling and how your breath feels as it enters and leaves your body. Pause here. Follow your breath. Now, notice a thought or experience that is troubling you. It might be a physical experience, such as a painful back or a headache. It might be a thought, such as "I'm cold," "I don't like to meditate," "I'm stressed out today," or "My marriage is in trouble." Shift your focus from your breath to this thought or experience. Pause here. Now, imagine if this thought or experience was its own entity. What color or colors would it be? What shape is it? What texture? Focus there. Take a good look at it. Now, imagine it leaving your body and floating out to the middle of the room. Take a look at it out there. Is it different having it out in the middle of the room? Now, allow it to grow. Let it get bigger and denser and more vibrant in color. Take a moment to look at it. Pause here. Now, imagine you are walking around it like a piece of sculpture. Study it with a curious mind. Take however long you like to visualize walking around this object. Now, imagine it getting smaller. As it gets smaller, it also becomes lighter. Lighter in density, lighter in color, lighter in weight. It continues to get smaller and lighter. Smaller and lighter. Smaller and lighter . . . until it becomes so small and so light that it floats back to you and lands on your shoulder, where you will carry it for the rest of the day.

Eight Favorite Examples of Common Defusion Techniques

1. Treat your thoughts like windows that pop up on your computer screen. Simply acknowledge them by "clicking" them to close them, or click the "minimizing" tab (the "–") to allow them to remain present while you shift your attention to the task you are engaged in on the primary screen.

2. Notice that your thoughts are the exhaust of your life, rather than the engine or steering wheel, by picturing your thoughts, emotions, and physical sensations exiting an exhaust pipe. Notice that sometimes when you hit the accelerator, the exhaust may increase in thickness, odor, and darkness. Try not to take the perspective that you are driving away from these internal experiences as they exit the exhaust pipe. Rather, try to experience this as a part of the natural course of everyday life.

3. Use the following language templates to gain distance from your thoughts, while allowing them to be.

   - "I'm having the thought that _____" (e.g., "I'm having the thought that I'm a loser").
   - "I'm having the emotion of _____ and the judgment that _____" (e.g., "I'm having the emotion of sadness and the judgment that this makes me weak).
   - "I'm having the sensation of _____ and the thought that _____" (e.g., "I'm having the sensation of a pounding heart and the thought that I might be having a heart attack").

4. Repeat your troublesome thoughts in a funny or peculiar voice. For example, say "I'm a loser" repeatedly in Daffy Duck's voice until you experience the thought differently, and perhaps experience some "air" with respect to it.

5. Sing your thoughts to the melody of your favorite song. For example, you could sing "Oh God, I've ruined my day" to the tune of Britney Spears's "Oops, I Did It Again."

6. Observe your thoughts as you would observe players at an athletic event while you're sitting in the audience looking down at the field.

7. Imagine that your challenging thoughts were connected to and contained in a physical object like a pen or your keys. Whenever the troubling thought pops into your head, remember the location of the object, such as touching your pocket to feel that the keys are there. You can remind yourself, "Yes, I still have these thoughts."

8. "Thanking the mind." Treat your mind as an external being that just keeps generating solutions to problems, visions of potential threats, and critical evaluations, because that is just what it does naturally, like a fish swims or a bird flies. In a sense, your mind is just doing the job it was given by nature. When you notice the troubling thoughts, you can simply say "Thanks, mind, for bringing these thoughts. It's all good, though. I've got this. Thanks for doing your job."

Self-Reflective Questions

Now that you have had the opportunity to practice noticing thoughts that get in your way as you try to move through your life in meaningful ways, take a moment to reflect on what you can take away from these experiences. What has your experience of defusion been?

_____

_____

_____

_____

_____

_____

_____

_____

_____

_____

_____

_____

Have you noticed any particular patterns of thoughts that keep you stuck or lead to avoidance? If so, what were they?

_____

_____

_____

_____

_____

_____

_____

_____

_____

_____

_____

_____

How do you understand the influence of fusion/defusion on the problem area you are working with in this workbook? How might this realization influence your actions moving forward?

_____

_____

_____

_____

_____

_____

_____

_____

_____

_____

_____

_____

_____

Can you remember a time when you were particularly fused during a session? The next time this happens, what will you do differently?

_____

_____

_____

_____

_____

_____

_____

_____

_____

_____

_____

_____

_____

_____

Have you learned anything new about your work as a therapist from this module? If so, what?

_____

_____

_____

_____

_____

_____

_____

_____

_____

_____

_____

_____

Acceptance

As you come to understand and cultivate psychological flexibility, you will gain a deeper, more experiential knowing of what we mean by "acceptance" in ACT. In this workbook, we use both the term *acceptance* and the term *willingness* to describe the dimension of psychological flexibility that points to our ability to acknowledge the nature of our experience in the moment, whatever it may be, and to remain open and available to the fullness of this experience, as much as we can. This knowing includes an appreciation and experience of openness and nonelaborative awareness of the here and now. It implies an ability to broaden our ground of experiencing and to make space for our experience in the present moment. It involves a choice to be with things as they are—hence the utility of the "will" in "willingness." The importance and meaning of acceptance in ACT is reflected in the name of this therapy and found in the first half of our definition of psychological flexibility: "contacting the present moment as a conscious human being, fully and without needless defense" (Hayes et al., 2012, p. 96). Acceptance and willingness are beyond dispositions—they are active processes—actions we can take rather than outcomes that remain. When we choose to be accepting in response to our experiences, we are choosing to be willing to have the reality of our private events as they are, in a given moment, without trying to change or avoid them.

Practicing experiential acceptance requires an understanding of how your thoughts and feelings influence your behavior, how your mind works in response to pain, and how you have learned to respond to your experiences. This insight into the true nature of cognitions and affect allows us new perspectives and new ways of being with our experience. We can come to understand transient mental events as they are, not as a direct reflection of reality or the self.

For therapists, a willingness to accept vulnerable feelings that arise during our sessions can be challenging. We are all vulnerable to the pull of EA and subject to the same language-based problem-solving techniques inherent in human cognition. Thus, the countermeasures of acceptance and willingness become core experiential processes in ACT, for both therapist and client. In this module, you get in touch with and cultivate your willingness and capacity for acceptance in service of your values and valued aims. We offer some exercises throughout to assist you in having a deeper understanding of getting at the core processes of acceptance and willingness. These exercises guide you through the skills and practice of acceptance and willingness through self-practice, which are followed by written self-reflection questions. By engaging in these activities, you get a firsthand understanding of what you will ask of yourself, as well as ask of your clients, in therapy. The more willing you are to engage in this core process, the more you will be able to understand how to apply this in your own life, as well as in the therapy room.

Getting to Know Acceptance and Willingness

In ACT, acceptance is understood as a behavior, a skill you can learn and practice. It involves *active receptivity and curiosity* about your experience. This process begins with a nonelaborative awareness of ever-changing experiences as they arise. These behaviors or skills require practice and a change in the way that we view our experiences and perceptions (Hayes & Feldman, 2004). These observed experiences include sensations, thoughts, emotions, and other responses to our experiences in the world. Acceptance, then, *is the practice of just letting these things be and experiencing them as they are*. It involves the *willingness to feel what you are feeling, think what you are thinking, and allowing yourself to acknowledge these experience as they occur* (Hayes, 2005).

Willingness is often used to help understand the meaning of acceptance in ACT. The aim here is to emphasize the active practice and disposition included in acceptance processes (Westrup, 2014). These processes, being accept*ing* and will*ing*, are actively cultivated and engaged in the service of openness to the here and now. This is not a passive decision and is different from "tolerating" or "wallowing" in the occurrence of our painful experiences (Batten, 2011). When we choose willingness, we choose to engage with the totality of our experience. This form of acceptance can provide new ways of attending to undesirable or unwanted experiences, providing alternatives to engaging in habitual or dysfunctional patterns, such as avoidance (Hayes & Shenk, 2004). As we will see, acceptance and willingness processes are in opposition to effortful control and the alternative to EA (Luoma et al., 2007). While acceptance gives us more options to responding to our painful private events and freedom to move toward our values, EA limits our choices and often leaves our lives feeling smaller, less in line with our values.

EA Undermines Flexibility

As discussed, EA represents our attempts to ignore, avoid, or control our experiences, often despite any long-term behavioral difficulties or unintended consequences of these attempts (Hayes et al., 2012). These consequences often come in the form of amplifying our pain and struggle. When we try to escape difficult or painful private events, they become more salient, and tend to increase in their intensity and frequency (Marcks & Woods, 2005; Wegner, 1994; Wenzlaff & Wegner, 2000). These unintended consequences reflect the paradox of trying to suppress or control our private experiences: "If you are not willing to have it, you will" (Hayes, 2005).

This tendency to engage in EA is baked into the function and our use of human language. Over the course of our lives, we develop rules about which experiences are acceptable and which are not and we learn to avoid the experiences we deem unacceptable. This strategy is a helpful approach to problem solving for our external world and physical events that occur around us, but not within us. When we recognize a problem in our environment, we can come up with ways to solve it, change it, or avoid it, and then take the appropriate actions to do so. For instance, if you noticed that it started raining and your windows were open, and you didn't want the rain to come inside, you would naturally get up and close the windows. As we mentioned above, this is not the case for our private events, however. The more we attempt to avoid them, the stronger they become.

EA strategies, such as emotion or thought suppression, are commonly used in reaction to disturbing or unpleasant thoughts, feelings, or urges (Hayes et al., 1996). These strategies not only can be negatively reinforcing but they also limit our options, making our lives feel smaller. When we are fused with our thinking, or engaged in emotional reasoning, we take thoughts as literal and our feelings as indicators of truth—they are believed and our behavior is shaped in response to this take on "reality." For instance, if you are nervous about an upcoming public talk, your mind might produce thoughts like "Everyone is going to laugh at me" or "Who do I think I am to give this talk? I'm an imposter!" You might try to distract yourself and ignore or challenge these thoughts. The more you try not to think about these things, the more distressing the whole process may seem. Perhaps you might avoid working on your talk or cancel the talk altogether. The following exercise involves two thought experiments to help illuminate the difference between control and willingness approaches to our cognitions, and is adapted from *Get Out of Your Mind and Into Your Life* (Hayes, 2005).

✍ EXERCISE. "Don't Have That Thought" and "Have Any Thought"

For this exercise, you will use and track a challenging thought in two different thought experiments: one focuses on *control* and one focuses on *willingness*. You will be instructed to engage with your thinking and track the frequency of your challenging thought throughout these two experiments. To complete these exercises, you will need a watch or timer and the following form to guide you.

To begin, pick a thought that you struggle with, one that is involved with your suffering. Choose one of the thoughts that is involved with the problem area you have been working with throughout this workbook. While there may be many thoughts presenting themselves to you as you begin, pick one discrete, challenging thought or phrase that comes to mind and write it in the following blank:

Over the course of the last week, about how many times did this thought show up
(if you are unsure, make an educated guess)? _____

Now, let's use and track that thought in two different thought experiments: first, one of control—"Don't have that thought"—and second, one of willingness—"Have any thought."

1. **DON'T HAVE THAT THOUGHT.** Take out a watch or timer and prepare to time yourself for the next 5 minutes. Also take out a pencil and piece of paper and position them so that you can make a small "tick" mark, check, or X on the paper, even with your eyes closed. When you are ready, begin the timer, close your eyes, and try not to have that thought. You can use any and all of your avoidance strategies—just remember, your aim is to suppress or block thinking about the thought you have chosen to avoid. Whenever you have the thought, mark the paper.

   Once the 5 minutes are up, look at your piece of paper and count the marks to record how many times that thought showed up while you were trying not to have it. How many times did the thought pop into your head? _____

2. **HAVE ANY THOUGHT.** For the next exercise, you will again use a watch or timer and prepare to time yourself for the next 5 minutes. Use your pencil and the other side of your piece of paper, and, again, position them so that you can make a small "tick" mark, check, or X on the paper, even with your eyes closed. When you are ready, begin the timer, close your eyes, and *allow your mind to have any thought it wishes to have*. Wherever your mind goes, just let it go there. Allow yourself to think as you wish. If the thought you had chosen earlier pops up, just make a mark on the paper.

   When these 5 minutes are up, record how many times you had that thought while thinking about anything you wanted or occurred to you. _____

Now, take a few moments to reflect on these experiences. What did you notice? When you tried to not have the thought, what happened? And when you allowed yourself to have any thought, what happened?

Compounding Pain through Avoidance: Turning Pain into Suffering

One of us (Joann) gave an example of what it feels like to be running late for a client, and how that can illustrate the relationships among pain, avoidance, and suffering. Imagine a therapist who is driving to her office, and begins to face some unavoidable traffic. When this happened, Joann had been living with cancer and facing some challenges in her life, and she felt like she had been struggling around the edges of professional responsibilities, sometimes being a few minutes late for sessions. Imagine the very moment she realizes she will definitely be late for her client, knowing that this will be distressing for both of them. Earlier, she had difficulty getting out of the house on time, dealing with family and work. She slipped out with barely enough time left to get in the door just as her session would start, and now she's stuck in traffic. She can't turn around, and she can't take another route. She is at a dead stop and can't do anything about it. Her frustration and her anger with herself was already high, fueled by fusion with her thoughts about competency/incompetency. Now, this traffic jam feels like "the last straw." Joann starts tearing up. She pounds her steering wheel with her fists while yelling "No! No! No!" She tells herself that this can't be happening. Her palms start sweating and her breath becomes short. Perhaps this is an understandable upwelling of anger and shame. But is the traffic moving any faster for her? Does the struggle against the experience help her to bear the distress any more effectively? Through lack of acceptance of the situation, Joann has allowed her pain to transform into suffering. Like so many of us, so much of the time, rather than acknowledging the inherent stress in the situation, riding the waves of emotion, and taking whatever actions were available, Joann found herself struggling, suffering, and experiencing helplessness.

ACT acknowledges that pain is not a choice for us. If we are alive, we will experience pain. The more we rail against this reality, the more it will assert its presence. The more we try to fight it, the more it fights back. The reality of human pain is inevitable. Suffering, however, results from our sometimes invisible choice to try and avoid internal pain. Joann was in pain while sitting in the traffic, knowing she would be late for her session. The more she fought that reality, the more suffering ensued. Her response to this, pounding on the steering wheel, was, in a sense, a choice. It likely resulted in more tension, and possibly sore hands. She might have chosen to sit in the moment with the traffic, willing to have the experience and accepting that life was not going the way she wanted. She could have come to terms with the fact that her client might be hurt, disappointed, or angry. In the reality of this context, she could have chosen a values-consistent way to respond, perhaps pulling over to contact the client, alert her client to the situation, apologize, and offer a gesture of repair. She might have practiced some self-forgiveness and self-kindness consciously. When she chose to struggle against the reality of the situation and the texture of her emotional response, Joann forfeited her freedom of action, and suffering ensued.

The paradigm of compounding our pain into suffering through EA is nicely summarized in the following metaphorical equation:

$$PAIN + AVOIDANCE = SUFFERING$$
$$SUFFERING > PAIN$$

As the level of EA increases, so does the degree of suffering. Suffering then becomes "greater than" the pain. ACT posits that, while you can't choose how much pain you have in your life, you can choose some of the degree of your suffering. In the next section, you will have a chance to look at the ways in which you attempt to avoid or control some of your painful private events.

The Behaviors and Consequences of EA

While we are busy attempting to avoid, suppress, or control our unpleasant private experiences, we lose contact with what is happening right here, right now. Our lives, values, and committed actions can be left on the sidelines while we engage in the work of suppressing what we don't want to think or feel. So, it seems there is a high price to pay for avoiding our painful private experiences—increased suffering and a lack of contact with those things that give our lives a sense of meaning, purpose, and vitality.

So, what does EA look like? There are many ways in which we attempt to avoid, alter, or control our private experiences. Russ Harris (2009) has summarized ways that we can avoid or overcontrol our experiences as "D.O.T.S." as in "joining the dots":

- **D**istraction.
- **O**pting out of activities.
- "**T**hinking strategies"—like worry, rumination, and overthinking.
- **S**ubstance misuse.

The use of strategies for avoiding, suppressing, or controlling private events often comes at the cost of valued living. What price have you paid for EA? What have you been busy doing in response to your painful thoughts and feelings? Take a moment to reflect on those strategies you have adopted to deal with painful private events and what it has cost you. What are those things you do that keep you busy avoiding, rather than living? The following exercise will help you bring awareness to those private events you typically respond to with EA and the consequences, indented or unintended, of these responses.

EXERCISE. What I'm Doing When I Am Avoiding and What It Has Cost Me

The worksheet on page 165 is intended to help you create an inventory of your experientially avoidant strategies and their consequences. Emphasize the problem area you have chosen for this workbook as you engage with this exercise. In the first column, list some of the painful private events that you attempt to avoid or control. Then, in the second column, list those things you do to get rid of, fix, or ignore these experiences. Next, evaluate the effectiveness of these strategies: How have they worked for you? Finally, note the costs and unintended consequences of engaging in these strategies. Dennis's example appears on the following page.

EXAMPLE. Dennis's EA Strategies

Painful private events (thoughts, feelings, or sensations)	What I do to avoid, suppress, or control these experiences	How much have avoidance, suppression, and control strategies worked for me?	What's the cost of using these strategies? What are the unintended consequences?
Despair, feeling overwhelmed, feeling incompetent.	Compulsively scheduling, working, and making lists.	Mostly hasn't worked. Still, some of the basic organization tasks are important when they aren't compulsive.	More time spent in struggling to organize work than in getting things done or enjoying life.
Asking myself how I can ever manage to change my behavior and feel more capable.	Waking up an hour earlier than needed, worrying and ruminating.	Only leads to anxiety and inactivity for the period lost to overthinking	Poor sleep, enhanced anxiety, time lost in the morning that could be spent in meditation, music practice, or exercise.
Self-criticism, cruel evaluation of all of my inadequacies, inner critic raging.	Distraction from work by taking long breaks and getting lost looking things up on the Internet or playing video games.	Time is neither spent in valued action, nor in constructive self-care. I feel I "need a break" but only wind up feeling worse.	My inner critic feels justified in being abusive, time is wasted, slower progress toward meaningful goals.
Anxiety about how life will change for the worse if every detail isn't taken care of.	Taking time away from friends and hobbies to work on projects, but then feeling exhausted, burnt out, sleeping, or binge-watching TV.	This does result in some work being done, but far less than if it were in manageable doses and balanced with self-care.	Relationships suffer, burnout and tiredness gets in the way of exercise and activities of self-realization.
Sadness in feeling isolated and overworked. Feeling alone and lonely.	Shopping on the Internet or Ebay for musical equipment, overeating, and ruminating.	Briefly feel like I am doing something meaningful, then a crash of isolation and sadness.	Financial drain, struggling with being overweight, increased anxiety.

EXERCISE. My EA Strategies

Painful private events (thoughts, feelings, or sensations)	What I do to avoid, suppress, or control these experiences	How much have avoidance, suppression, and control strategies worked for me?	What's the cost of using these strategies? What are the unintended consequences?

From Recognition to Acceptance to Action

Even if we acknowledge the suffering that results from our attempts at avoidance, moving from unwillingness to acceptance of pain is not an easy process. The thought "If I can just rid my mind of these thoughts, the pain will go away," is an attractive one. Again, we've been taught this message many times in many forms throughout our lives: "Don't worry"; "You've got to get over this"; "Just don't think about it"; "Do something to distract yourself." When we were raised, we were far more likely to hear this kind of advice than to be told to take an observer's perspective on our thoughts and cultivate the willingness to have them.

As noted earlier, avoidance works very well in our external environment. We realize that we can close the window when it is raining and not get wet. Our human capacity for symbolic representation through language allows us to have private experiences that "feel like the real world," and so it would only make sense that we apply the same problem-solving approach to this inner representation of our world. Avoidance of mental events can also seem to work in the short term—that is, we get some relief, albeit brief relief. This kind of negative reinforcement provides enough "workability," or relief, that we keep relying on this strategy.

Imagine running barefoot on a hot, sandy beach. When you come to stop, you notice the sand beneath you is very hot, scalding the soles of your feet. Instead of continuing to move over the sand, you stop and pour cool water over your feet. Initially, you would experience relief, but over time, the water evaporates, the sand becomes increasingly hot, scorching your feet all over again, and so you reach for more water, repeating this cycle. Until, that is, you run out of water and ultimately, never complete your run. You might even find yourself carrying more and more water with you, each time you go for a run on the beach, rather than accepting that the sand on the beach will be hot and no amount of water can change that. Maybe you accept this nature of hot sand, go for a run in the woods, or bring some running shoes.

This is how EA hooks us—the brief relief of escape or control keeps us reaching for the water, only delaying the inevitable return of heat and pain, perhaps even making us more sensitive to its return, feeling hotter than ever before. This is how avoidance can be negatively reinforcing, by providing short-term escape from threatening material and distressing physical sensations, it takes away the heat, but only in the short term. In the long term, however, EA helps maintain painful thoughts or images, inhibiting emotional processing and ultimately keeps us stuck in a perpetual cycle of avoidance (Huppert & Alley, 2004; Mathews, 1990).

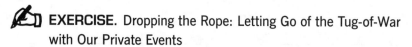 **EXERCISE.** Dropping the Rope: Letting Go of the Tug-of-War with Our Private Events

When we are suffering, it can feel as if we are in a tug-of-war with our thoughts, feelings, and even our bodily sensations. The following classic exercise (Hayes et al., 1999) helps us to directly experience this tension and our fruitless attempts at avoiding our experiences.

There are many different variations and ways of using the tug-of-war exercise. Whether it is used as a therapeutic metaphor, guided imagery, or experiential exercise, the focus of the exercise is to demonstrate the effectiveness of "letting go" of the struggle with the private events, such as our thoughts that are trying to pull us off course from our value-laden life. The aim in this exercise is to come back to the present moment and to let go of struggling with private events.

We all inevitably find ourselves tugging on the other end of the rope from time to time. The emphasis here is not to avoid the rope but to increase awareness of when you have picked up the rope, to highlight your options in this experience, and to have the experience of letting go. It is a good idea to choose thoughts or feelings that involve the problem area you have been working through in this workbook, as you engage with the following exercise.

To prepare for this exercise in a group or pair format you may want to have a piece of rope or a twisted towel to use for a physical, experiential demonstration. As the tug-of-war is described, two partners can pull back and forth on the same physical object to simulate the inner struggle. If you are practicing this yourself, this technique can be conducted as an imagery exercise, or you could even tie a towel or cord to a furniture post, doorknob, or anchoring point to simulate an immovable tug-of-war. The following instructions can be recorded so that you might practice as a guided meditation. You can also download an audio version of this practice from the book's website (see the box at the end of the table of contents), or alternatively, you can read and memorize the following as guidelines for silent practice. You can use the following script and questions as a guide through this experiential practice.

The struggle we find ourselves in with our painful private events can feel like an endless game of tug-of-war. On the other end of the rope is a very strong opponent, one that you may know very well or that may be a new challenger. New or old, your opponent is the physical representation or metaphor for those private events you are struggling with currently. It could be your self-doubt, inner critic, feelings of depression or anxiety, physical pain, or anything that is getting in the way of your valued living. Take a moment and imagine what your opponent looks like. Recall what this part of you that you struggle with says to you. How does it feel? What form would it take? What size would it be? What facial expression would it make? What tone of voice would it use? When you are ready, answer the following written questions.

What are you currently struggling with? What does this opponent on the other side of the rope represent for you?

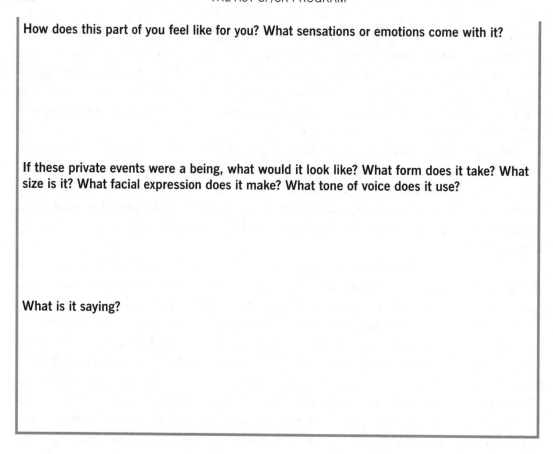

How does this part of you feel like for you? What sensations or emotions come with it?

If these private events were a being, what would it look like? What form does it take? What size is it? What facial expression does it make? What tone of voice does it use?

What is it saying?

Now, using this image of the painful private event that you have created, imagine you are in a tug-of-war with you on one end and the physical representation of your pain on the other. Just like your other private events, this opponent cannot touch you, but can say and act in ways that make you want to win this tug-of-war. The being on the other end of the rope says the painful words that you have aimed to avoid or shut out. In order to overcome them and make them go away, you need to win this tug-of-war, as far as you can tell. And when you begin to pull on the rope, your opponent pulls back, and it is as strong as you are. It is trying just as hard as you and always meets you with resistance. It isn't going anywhere, it seems.

At times your opponent is overbearing, and it may feel as if you are not strong enough. You are at risk of losing, or being stuck with this opponent forever. There may be other times when you might think you are overcoming the struggle, and winning. You might just pull hard enough to end the war, getting rid of it all together. As this struggle continues, the harder you pull, the harder your opponent pulls. So, you go on trying, pulling harder, digging in your heels, getting a stronger grip on the rope, pulling harder, and hopefully beating your opponent. You pull and pull, to no avail, nothing you try is working. And so it goes, seemingly unending, as you keep pulling back. You simply cannot overcome and get rid of this opponent. It isn't going anywhere. It seems the harder you pull, the stronger it is and it doesn't seem to ever tire out.

Now, bring your attention to how this experience feels. What does it feel like for you in this tug-of-war? What do you notice in your body? Your breathing? Body temperature? Facial expressions? What does it feel like to be in this struggle and to hear things like [use the examples]? Where is your attention focused? What thoughts show up? Perhaps you might notice the thought that maybe you might win this time, or that you might be stuck in this struggle forever or that your opponent will win. What else do you notice? What do you feel like doing?

On the one hand, you could pull harder, fight back more. Have you ever succeeded in getting rid of this opponent forever? How has all of this been working so far? What else could you do? What other choice do you have? Do you have to win this tug-of-war? What would happen if you were to stop fighting with this part of your experience? What if you decided to opt out of this tug-of-war and drop the rope?

Now, if you are willing, see whether you can try this option. Drop the rope.

Imagine what it might be like if you let go of the rope, letting it fall to the ground. What do you notice? What is different? Allow yourself to notice how this experience feels in your body. What does it feel like for you to drop the rope? Notice any changes in your muscles, breathing, body posture, and facial expressions. How do your hands and feet feel? You may notice that your hands and feet are no longer engaged—they are free for use as you choose. What would it mean if you were to not drop the rope? What would become available to you?

As you let go of the rope, you drop the impossible task of getting rid of your opponent. Your opponent has not disappeared, and it does not mean you have won. Your opponent is still there on the other end of the rope as its always been, taunting you, trying to get you to reengage. Perhaps your opponent is even judging you for dropping the rope in the first place. But in dropping the rope, you get to choose not to fight, not to pick up the rope, to turn toward your values instead, and do something perhaps more important to you.

When you dropped the rope, what did you notice? What did it feel like? Did you notice any changes in your muscles, breathing, body posture, and facial expressions? How did your hands and feet feel?

What did the experience of dropping the rope mean for you? What would become available to you?

 EXAMPLE: Joann's Responses to Dropping the Rope

What are you currently struggling with? What does this opponent on the other side of the rope represent for you?
On the other side of the rope is doubt. Doubt regarding my abilities to open a private practice. I often struggle with doubt when I am trying to move forward in my career. I doubt my capacity as a businessperson and as a private practitioner. Doubt is trying to pull me away from opening a new practice.

If these private events were a being, what would it look like?
A snarling beast, with large hands and feet. It makes a scowling face with a strong glare in its dark eyes. It is very large and strong, and very loud at times, with a deep, booming voice.

What is it saying?

It tells me that I have no idea what I am doing. I don't know how to run a private practice. I don't know anything about billing, or HIPAA laws, or how much I should charge with my license, or billing codes. It says I'm going to fail, that I can't do this. It tells me that I'm being naïve by opening a private practice before I am sure that I can accomplish these things. Other people who open private practices know more than me. That I might fail, go bankrupt, and let my family down.

When you dropped the rope, what did you notice? What did it feel like? Did you notice any changes in your muscles, breathing, body posture, and facial expressions? How did your hands and feet feel?

Dropping the rope was hard at first, I really want to defeat my doubt. But then when I dropped the rope, there was a sort of release, a freedom. I felt lighter, less tension. My whole body felt like it was mine again, that I was free to be, I didn't have to fight. I could use my hands and feet, they were no longer braced with tension and struggle. They were free, I felt free, like I could choose how I wanted to be and what I wanted to do.

What did the experience of dropping the rope mean for you? What would become available to you?

If I drop the rope with doubt, I will take more steps to open my private practice. It might not be perfect, and perhaps I won't have all the answers. I will question myself from time to time and I can get support and guidance from organizations and colleagues. I might make mistakes, but I'm willing to keep learning and find my way. It's better than not trying at all.

Acceptance Is Not about Seeking Comfort or Amplifying Pain

A common misconception of acceptance is that it will eventually lead to greater comfort or greater suffering. The aim of acceptance practice in ACT is neither about feeling better, or for that matter, feeling worse (Hayes, 2005). Those are not our aims. Remember that the acceptance pillar of ACT is referred to as the *open* pillar and involves a receptivity to what is. It's not about feeling more or less than what is already present in our current experience. It is a willingness toward all experiences—even unwanted ones. In fact, acceptance is not a feeling at all (Westrup, 2014). Instead, it can be viewed as an intentional stance; a willingness to move through and with the discomfort and move toward a purposeful, vital life. Therefore, understanding one's intention in this practice is important. If our aim is to get rid of our pain through acceptance, then it's not acceptance, and as we will see, it is not moving us toward our valued aims.

EXERCISE. Tracking Opportunities to Practice Willingness and Acceptance

The following record is intended to help you bring awareness to acceptance and willingness practices. These experiences can be formal (planned practice or exercises) or informal (as opportunities that arise for practicing acceptance throughout your day-to-day experiences).

Date	What was the situation? What were you willing to experience in that moment?	How did you practice or choose acceptance in that moment?	What did you notice?

LAURA'S EXAMPLE

Date	What was the situation? What were you willing to experience in that moment?	How did you practice or choose acceptance in that moment?	What did you notice?
4/14	Yoga class. I usually push myself a bit hard at times and sometimes get frustrated when my knees start to bother me. This week I practiced accepting these experiences as they arose and accepting my limits and capabilities.	I used this yoga class as an opportunity to practice accepting my limits, simply noticing when I felt frustrated or a willingness to listen to my body and go with my flow, in the moment.	I felt a bit more encouraged and yoga felt more "doable" with this kind of approach. I was less distracted, in a way, less in my head. I may have even enjoyed it more, even though the frustrations showed up.
4/16	I hit my "funny bone" getting ready to leave for work this morning. I noticed the pain and used it as an opportunity to practice.	Instead of ignoring it or berating myself for being clumsy, I somehow remembered the practice of letting pain be pain and not compounding that pain through unwillingness and avoidance.	It hurt. I do not like hitting my elbow like that. Nobody does. But I really noticed the difference between other experiences like this when I made it worse when I was not willing to accept that I hurt myself in the first place.
4/18	Saw that a former classmate published a paper in a peer-reviewed journal and began doubting myself and thinking that I am not doing enough.	Chose to accept the thought "I'm not doing enough" rather than avoiding the thought. I imagined dropping the rope and turning toward the next steps in my private practice work.	By being more willing and choosing to accept the doubt thoughts, I was freer to work on things that mattered to me. And there was room for more of my experience. I also felt happy for her and sent her a quick congrats email, which felt more in line with my relationship values, too.

An allegory that's been part of the ACT community for many years to help illustrate the ineffectiveness of the control agenda is the man-in-a-hole metaphor.

 Self-Reflective Questions

What was your experience as you engaged in the acceptance and willingness exercises? What observations were most vivid to you in this module?

_____

_____

_____

_____

_____

_____

_____

_____

_____

_____

_____

_____

What was different in these experiences from your everyday responses to painful thoughts and feelings?

_____

_____

_____

_____

_____

_____

_____

_____

_____

_____

_____

Was there anything in these experiences you would like to remember?

_____

_____

_____

_____

_____

_____

_____

_____

_____

_____

_____

_____

_____

How do you plan to practice acceptance and willingness skills going forward?

_____

_____

_____

_____

_____

_____

_____

_____

_____

_____

_____

_____

_____

How do you plan to integrate acceptance and willingness practice into your clinical practice?

_____

_____

_____

_____

_____

_____

_____

_____

_____

_____

_____

_____

_____

SECTION D

ENGAGED

MODULE 10

Values Authorship

Take a moment and consider the following questions: What is most important to you in life? How do you value being in the world? What gives your life meaning and purpose? These questions are substantial and we sometimes don't take the time to explicitly answer them. In the rush and demands of our everyday lives and the pull of our private events, it is easy to lose contact with what matters the most to us. Imagine embarking on a journey without first specifying your destination or means of travel. It wouldn't make sense or be very effective. Yet, many of us live our lives in precisely this way. We show up to life as passive passengers, following rules and situational demands, and all too often, we let our private experiences dictate the direction and shape our lives take. Becoming the author of one's values puts us back in charge of our journey, clarifying the directions we move in or return to when we get sidetracked. Without the direction that values point us in, we are likely to spend a good deal of our time on earth avoiding painful thoughts and feelings. When we clarify our values, the ways in which we want to be in the world, and choose to rely on our values as guidance, we are freed up to behave in ways that are dictated by these values rather than basing our lives on the feelings we would rather avoid, and which feeling states we would like to chase.

Becoming an author of one's values is essential in cultivating psychological flexibility and in living a vital life. In this way, ACT SP/SR invites us to consciously author valued aims. This involves increasing our awareness of what matters most, and also learning how to embody those values. Together, we explore this process and deepen your understanding of values clarification in ACT and in your SP/SR work.

Why Values Matter

Values are inherently related to our suffering. Experiences of pain and suffering are often connected to something we care deeply about. As Steve Hayes (2016) said in his TEDx Nevada talk on turning pain into purpose, "We care where we hurt and we hurt where we care." Those things we tend to criticize ourselves about or have the potential for the most meaningful losses are related to our values. Ask yourself, What are some of the things that I criticize myself about most? Now consider the following: What would you have to stop caring about for this to no longer cause you suffering? For example, if you criticize yourself for not being as involved and caring as you could be as a parent, what would you have to stop caring about in order to not feel an urge to criticize yourself? Would you have to stop caring about how effectively and lovingly you parent? Are you willing to stop caring about that? Could you even stop caring about that? For most of us, the answer is no, of course not. These issues are often connected to things that matter the most in our lives. In ACT, we sometimes say, *In your pain you find your values, and in your values you find your pain* (Hayes & Lillis, 2012). In fact, part of what gives the process of acceptance so much power in our ACT work is the way that we look inside painful experiences to discover depth and meaning. We can then live toward that meaning, carrying the pain of the human condition as a part of the wholeness of our experience.

Values clarification in ACT has been said to involve increasing one's awareness of the "sweetness" in one's life (Wilson & DuFrene, 2009), even when this means contacting pain and sometimes grief. In this way, our pain and values can arrive hand in hand. Increased awareness of what we care about can also lead to awareness of blocks to progress or to remembered and feared losses. For some, values work may bring to mind times when we haven't lived in accordance with our values. Sometimes such experiences invoke an acute awareness of our finality. It is important to be aware that these sorts of experiences can pull for psychologically inflexible responding. Determining your values isn't necessarily easy and may contain some unexpected distractors. Any difficulties you experience in this regard might be useful to consider during your self-reflection periods, so make a note of them.

The Dance between Valuing and Suffering

In ACT, the use of the term *values* refers to ongoing, evolving patterns of behaviors that are intrinsically reinforcing. In ACT SP/SR, as in all forms of ACT, values are considered personally constructed guidelines for meaningful ways of living one's life. In other words, values provide us with ways of being and doing in the world. Values are not rigid rules, nor subject to social manipulation (Luoma et al., 2007). These valued orientations are stable yet dynamic, able to grow and evolve with time and context (Batten, 2011).

Our values can help us shape and motivate our behavior in lasting ways. They point us toward what matters and in turn inform the process of creating values-based goals and engaging in committed actions. Because of their intrinsically reinforcing nature, our freely chosen values make the challenging work involved in ACT "worth it." They reinforce processes such as willingness and defusion, and are an essential component of psychological flexibility. Those things we value can inspire courage and motivation to move toward our valued aims.

Constructing and understanding values can also give meaning to the present moment. The ability to recognize what is significant in a given moment provides us with a choice: to continue one's current behavior or change that behavior in service of one's values and responding to a current context in meaningful and effective ways. This process involves flexible perspective taking and mindful awareness. When you contact the present moment, choice becomes available, and when you clarify your values, the opportunity for choosing valued informed decisions becomes more apparent. Thus, when we look at the definition of psychological flexibility, it becomes clear how necessary an understanding of one's values are. Without this awareness of choice in a given moment, intentional values-based behaviors can become more challenging and can lead to feeling stuck in old patterns of behavior and EA.

Values Are a Process, Not a Product

In ACT, values are considered as an ongoing process. They are orientations that do not contain endpoints. They are the routes, not the destinations. For example, one might value "being a loving father." One can always be more loving—that is, one never arrives at a concrete end known as "loving father." The value of "loving father" is not achieved or gotten, it is embodied as an ongoing behavioral process. In fact, being a loving father means behaving in loving ways, even in the absence of any feelings of love. In general, it's easy to behave lovingly when one is consumed with the feeling of love, but more challenging when it's absent and when other emotions are present (e.g., anger). Because emotions wax and wane, much like the weather, a changing emotional landscape is all but guaranteed. Our values, however, are stable and able to adapt with our changing lives and experiences. Therefore, what counts is our commitment to behaving lovingly independent of our current experience of love.

Goals or aims, in contrast to values, are actions that do contain concrete ends. These could include certain behaviors or ways of being or doing that embody one's values. For example, an individual living in accordance with their "loving father" value might work toward goals, such as reading a story with their child each night, leaving work early to attend their child's sporting event, or they might just spend unstructured time with their child each day. Goals, like values, exist in the realm of overt behavior, but unlike values, they involve achievable ends.

Values and goals work together. Values orient us, whereas goals provide feedback about how well we're living in relation to our values. Goals help us operationalize our values. As we begin, it's important in ACT for therapists and clients to understand the distinction between values and goals, so spend some time with the following exercise.

EXERCISE. Discriminating Goals from Values

Next to each item in the list below, write "G" if it is a goal and "V" if it is a value. Then check your answers against ours.

1. Exercise 3 days a week. _____
2. To live contentedly within my means. _____
3. Be a loving spouse. _____
4. Attend church weekly. _____
5. Take care of my body physically, mentally, and spiritually. _____
6. Practice mindfulness 20 minutes each day. _____
7. Live mindfully. _____
8. Be compassionate toward others. _____
9. Spend time engaged in my hobbies at least once per week. _____
10. Give out cards on my friends' birthdays. _____

Our answers:

1. This is a goal, because this has an achievable end. This goal may be tied to a value, such as "to be physically healthy," but it doesn't inherently reflect a quality of doing and being more than an end to be gained.
2. This is a value. This specifies a quality of action and a direction, with no concrete end.
3. This too is a value. One can never arrive at "loving spouse." One can always be more loving, and return to loving behavior, again and again.
4. This is a goal. Either one does or does not attend church each week.
5. This is a value. A direction is specified.
6. This is a goal. Can you say why? _____
7. This is a value. Can you say why? _____
8. This is a value. Can you say why? _____
9. This is a goal. Can you say why? _____
10. This is a goal. Can you say why? _____

Determining Your Values

Now that we have returned to the meaning of values work in ACT, let's take some time to reflect upon what matters most to us in our own lives. We continue by sitting with challenging questions, similar to the ones we asked at the beginning of this module, and even earlier in the imaginary eulogy exercise. These exercises ask, "How do you want to feel when you look back on your life?" and "How do you want to be remembered by those in your life?" The following imagery exercise guides you through questions about what is most important to you in different areas of your life, drawing from a range of classic ACT values authorship and experiential practices. When you have completed the experience, you will be given the opportunity to author your values in clearly verbally constructed ways, making your values more explicit in a written exercise.

EXERCISE. What Do I Want My Life to Stand For?

Before beginning, ensure that you are in a comfortable place with minimal distractions. The following guided instructions are for an imagery exercise that focuses on those areas in your life that are most important to you. After we establish our practice by centering in the present moment, you will be asked to bring to mind different areas of your life and then guided through a series of questions about what is most important to you in each area. Use your imagery skills, imagining what you might hear, see, and do in terms of your values from your first-person perspective. After each question, give yourself some time to sit with whatever arises, mindfully. As best you can, see whether you can allow yourself to come in contact with your experience in each moment of the following practice. You can download an audio version of this practice from the book's website (see the box at the end of the table of contents), or record yourself reading the instructions and play them back.

As you begin, allow your eyes to close. Now, gently direct your attention to the experience of breathing. Allowing your awareness to rest with your breath. Simply observing the breath's natural rhythm. Noticing each inhale and each exhale. If your mind wanders to other thoughts or sensations, gently notice this experience and return your attention back to the breath.

After a few mindful breaths, with your next natural inhale, bring to mind what and who is most important to you in terms of family. When it comes to being a family member, what do you want to stand for? What type of family member would you be? Allow yourself to spend a few moments considering what you want to stand for in each of your roles and relationships in your family. When you are ready, with your next exhale, let go of these questions about family and gently return your attention to breathing.

When you are ready, bring to mind who and what might be important to you when it comes to romantic relationships. What do you want to stand for when it comes to romance and intimacy? What kind of romantic or intimate partner do you want to be? See whether you can allow yourself to contact what qualities are most important to you in terms of romance or intimacy. When you are ready, with your next exhale, let go of these questions and gently return your attention to your breath.

With your next inhale, bring to mind who and what matters to you in terms of your friendships and social life. What do you want to stand for as a friend? How do you want to be toward your friends? How do you like to treat others in your life? Noticing whatever arises and spending a few moments contacting what matters most to you in terms of friendships and social relationships. When you are ready, with your next exhale, let go of these questions and return your awareness to your breathing.

After settling your attention with the breath, on the next inhale, bring to mind who and what is most important to you when it comes to work. What do you want to stand for in your work? How do you want to work in a meaningful way? Allow yourself to consider these questions and what you value most in terms of work. And when you are ready, with your next natural exhale, let go of these questions and return your attention to breathing.

With your next inhale, bring to mind who and what matters to you in terms of education and learning. What do you want to stand for as a student or learner? How do you want to be when it comes to education? What approach to learning feels meaningful for you? Simply noticing whatever arises and spending a few moments contacting what matters most to you in terms of education. When you are ready, with your next exhale, let go of these questions and return your awareness to mindfully breathing in and breathing out.

With your next inhale, bring to mind the area of recreation in your life. Who or what matters most to you in terms of fun and recreation? How do you want to be when you are at play? Take some time to consider what fun, play, or recreation mean to you. And when you are ready, on the next exhale, let go and return your focus to your mindful breathing.

After a few mindful breaths, bring to mind who and what is most important to you when it comes to health and wellness. What do you want to stand for in terms of your health and wellness? How do you want to be and do in this area of your life? What is meaningful participation in wellness for you? Give yourself some time to contact your health and wellness values. When you are ready, with your next available exhale, let go of these questions and return your attention to your experience of breathing.

On the next breath, begin to expand your awareness to include what you want to stand for in all of these areas of living: family, romance, friendships, work, learning, recreation, and health and wellness. Once you have spent some time with this and are ready to form an intention of completing this practice, gently allow your breathing and attention to return to the breath. Noticing the sensations of your breathing here and now, and when you feel ready, you can open your eyes.

In the next exercise, you will have the opportunity to clarify and write down your values in the areas of living we just explored. As you go through the exercise, keep the following guidelines in mind:

- Shoot for the stars! This is your life and no one else's. In a world where there are no barriers, what would you want it to stand for? What do you want to orient your life around?
- Word your values statement broadly so that it has the potential of capturing a large pattern of behavioral activity.
- Try to encapsulate the value in one sentence or a few words. This will be your "values statement."
- After you've written your values statement, ask yourself, "If no one ever knew I lived in this way, would I still have wanted to be about that?" You may also find it useful to use specific persons when you ask yourself this question (e.g., "If my parents never knew . . ."). You may find it useful to ask yourself different versions of this question (e.g., "If my parents knew . . ."; "If my kids knew . . ."; "If 'no one' knew . . ."). Ideally, you'd want to live in a way uncontrolled from how others view your accomplishments.

- Ask yourself this about your values statement: "If living this way never made me feel good, and maybe even made me feel bad in some ways, am I still satisfied that I lived this way?" While living in accordance with your values often produces feelings of contentment, they should not be done for this purpose because this is not a reliable metric nor the reason for living in this way.
- Here are some example values statements:
  - To be loving and compassionate toward all living things.
  - To engage in meaningful scientific work.
  - To have a positive impact on the suffering in the world.
  - Make self-care a priority.
  - Teach my kids, through my actions, how to show up to emotional pain.

EXERCISE. Values Assessment Inventory

Below you will find a list of major life domains. In each domain, write a sentence that captures what you want to stand for in a given area of your life. Provide three ratings next to each domain. The first rating is how important that valued domain is to you (note that these do not need to be rank ordered), the second is how effective you believe you were at living out this value over the last week, and the third rating is how present you have generally been when living out this value during the preceding week. All ratings are from 0 to 10, with 10 = the most you could imagine.

LIFE DOMAIN VALUES INVENTORY AND ASSESSMENT

Family

Importance: _____   **Effectiveness:** _____   **Presence:** _____

What is most important to me: _____

_____

What I want to stand for (values statement): _____

_____

Romance and Intimacy

Importance: _____   **Effectiveness:** _____   **Presence:** _____

What is most important to me: _____

_____

What I want to stand for (values statement): _____

_____

Friendships

Importance: _____   **Effectiveness:** _____   **Presence:** _____

What is most important to me: _____

_____

What I want to stand for (values statement): _____

_____

Career

Importance: _____   **Effectiveness:** _____   **Presence:** _____

What is most important to me: _____

_____

What I want to stand for (values statement): _____

_____

Education

Importance: _____   **Effectiveness:** _____   **Presence:** _____

What is most important to me: _____

_____

What I want to stand for (values statement): _____

_____

Recreation and Play

Importance: _____   **Effectiveness:** _____   **Presence:** _____

What is most important to me: _____

_____

What I want to stand for (values statement): _____

_____

Health and Wellness

Importance: _____   **Effectiveness:** _____   **Presence:** _____

What is most important to me: _____

_____

What I want to stand for (values statement): _____

_____

Other

Importance: _____   **Effectiveness:** _____   **Presence:** _____

What is most important to me: _____

_____

What I want to stand for (values statement): _____

Self-Reflective Questions

What was your experience of values identification like? What thoughts, emotions, memories, and bodily sensations did you notice?

_____

_____

_____

_____

_____

_____

_____

_____

_____

_____

_____

_____

Did you find any of the valued directions you expressed in "conflict" with one another—that is, did it seem that moving in one direction might interfere with your moving in another important direction? If so, how might you make use of the other processes to move through this?

_____

_____

_____

_____

_____

_____

_____

_____

_____

_____

_____

_____

Valued directions are foundationless—that is, they cannot be based on reasons, although reasons may be present. Stating valued directions is akin to throwing a stake in the ground and simply asserting "I value this." When you articulated your valued directions, were any reasons present? If so, was it difficult to disentangle from them? What shows up for you when you ponder your valued directions containing no foundation?

_____

_____

_____

_____

_____

_____

_____

_____

_____

_____

_____

_____

_____

If it's not in your behavior, it's not in your life. Private experiences—such as thoughts, emotions, memories, and bodily sensations—are the exhaust of your life. In contrast, your behavior, guided by your values, is the engine. In what ways is this notion similar or dissimilar to how you've historically thought about living your life? What about how you've historically assisted clients with living theirs?

_____

_____

_____

_____

_____

_____

_____

_____

_____

_____

_____

_____

Can you articulate at least one thing you might do differently with a client as a result of your experience with personal values authorship?

_____

_____

_____

_____

_____

_____

_____

_____

_____

_____

_____

_____

Commitment, Part I

Determining Goals and Barriers to Commitment

Committed action involves cultivating behavioral patterns that are consistent with one's freely chosen values (Hayes et al., 2012; Moran, Bach, & Batten, 2018). Now that you have had the opportunity to clarify and author your values in the previous module, it is time to determine your valued actions and address any barriers to these goals. Working through goals, actions, and barriers is where the majority of committed action work in ACT is focused.

In this module, we find a way to measure how effective you've been in living in accordance with what is personally meaningful, we examine whether your pattern of living changes over time, and we set effective values-based goals.

How Well Have You Been Living?

In the Values Assessment Inventory exercise in the previous module, you were asked to provide three ratings for each values statement: (1) how important each valued domain is to you, (2) how effectively you think you've lived out each domain during the preceding week, and (3) how present you think you were as you lived out each domain across the same time period. The latter two ratings rely on recall (i.e., thinking back on the preceding week and rendering a subjective rating). This is a useful starting point for getting a sense of how well you've been living. However, it is more useful for you to record these ratings in real time. So, in addition to your initial recall ratings, we'd like you to monitor these two valued areas of living daily for at least 1 week before embarking on any changes. For the next days, at the end of each day, think back on the previous hours, and taking all things into consideration, provide the three ratings of valued living for each domain. Initially, we recommend that you select just one domain to work on. This should be a domain that relates directly to the problem area with which you have been working. You'll be able to get to the other important areas of living later. Which valued domain you select is up to you, but you may find it helpful to select a domain you've rated high in importance but low in effectiveness and/or presence. Once you've made your selection, write the valued direction you chose to target in the following space.

Values-based action(s) that I am monitoring:

✍ **EXERCISE.** My Valued Action Self-Monitoring Form

Identify one valued aim to focus on and list it below. Then each evening, taking your entire day into consideration, record your effectiveness and presence ratings on a 0–10 scale, where 10 = most effective and most present. For your purposes, "effectiveness" may be understood as how effectively you were able to translate your values into committed action in this part of your life. "Presence" can be understood as how much you were able to contact the present moment and be mindful of your intentions and values in your life. You can continue this practice for days, weeks, and even months, and it is a good idea to graph your data weekly. Note: If monitoring more than one valued direction, then use one form per valued direction.

Weekly valued aims monitored (list valued actions statement here):

_____

_____

_____

Week: _____

Date: _____/_____/_____ Effectiveness rating (0–10): _____   Presence rating (0–10): _____

Date: _____/_____/_____ Effectiveness rating (0–10): _____   Presence rating (0–10): _____

Date: _____/_____/_____ Effectiveness rating (0–10): _____   Presence rating (0–10): _____

Date: _____/_____/_____ Effectiveness rating (0–10): _____   Presence rating (0–10): _____

Date: _____/_____/_____ Effectiveness rating (0–10): _____   Presence rating (0–10): _____

Date: _____/_____/_____ Effectiveness rating (0–10): _____   Presence rating (0–10): _____

Date: _____/_____/_____ Effectiveness rating (0–10): _____   Presence rating (0–10): _____

✍ **EXERCISE.** My Daily Self-Monitoring Graph

To make better use of the information you track, we recommend displaying it visually on a graph. We also recommend that you continue taking data and visually displaying them throughout your engagement with this workbook and program.

Plot your average daily effectiveness and presence ratings for the specified values using the two graphs below. There is room for up to 10 weeks: E = effectiveness (0–10), P = presence (0–10).

Weekly valued aims monitored:

_____

_____

_____

Effectiveness:

	Mon.	Tues.	Wed.	Thurs.	Fri.	Sat.	Sun.
E10							
9							
8							
7							
6							
5							
4							
3							
2							
E1							

Presence:

	Mon.	Tues.	Wed.	Thurs.	Fri.	Sat.	Sun.
P10							
9							
8							
7							
6							
5							
4							
3							
2							
P1							

Observations:

_____

_____

_____

_____

EXAMPLE: Dennis's Valued Action Self-Monitoring Form

Weekly valued aims monitored (list valued actions statement here):

Waking up between 5:00 and 6:00 A.M., practicing zazen, and having a period of

writing before moving on to administrative tasks. Engaging in this activity with

mindfulness, present-moment contact, and self-kindness, as much as I can.

Week: <u>August 13 through August 19</u>

Date: <u>08/13/2018</u>   Effectiveness rating (0–10): <u>>7</u>   Presence rating (0–10): <u>5</u>
Date: <u>08/14/2018</u>   Effectiveness rating (0–10): <u>5</u>   Presence rating (0–10): <u>8</u>
Date: <u>08/15/2018</u>   Effectiveness rating (0–10): <u>9</u>   Presence rating (0–10): <u>9</u>
Date: <u>08/16/2018</u>   Effectiveness rating (0–10): <u>3</u>   Presence rating (0–10): <u>6</u>
Date: <u>08/17/2018</u>   Effectiveness rating (0–10): <u>8</u>   Presence rating (0–10): <u>9</u>
Date: <u>08/18/2018</u>   Effectiveness rating (0–10): <u>10</u>   Presence rating (0–10): <u>9</u>
Date: <u>08/19/2018</u>   Effectiveness rating (0–10): <u>6</u>   Presence rating (0–10): <u>6</u>

 EXAMPLE: Dennis's Daily Self-Monitoring Graph

Weekly valued aims monitored:

Waking up between 5:00 and 6:00 A.M., practicing zazen, and having a period of

writing before moving on to administrative tasks. Engaging in this activity with

mindfulness, present-moment contact, and self-kindness, as much as I can.

Effectiveness:

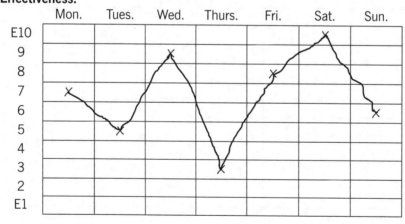

Presence:

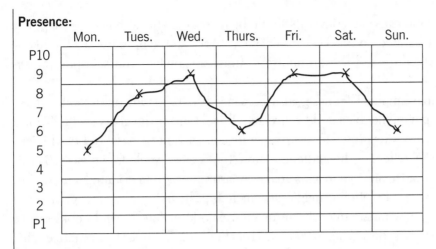

Observations:

There was a clear relationship between my ability to be consistent in getting out of bed

and sitting for a meditation practice and my ability to feel present and engaged with

my tasks each day. I was surprised by how much monitoring the activity helped with my

ability to commit.

Goals: Making Your Values Actionable

Now that you've specified your valued directions and identified one or two valued domains on which you would like to focus, it's time to articulate some goals tied to those values. Ultimately, however, living in accordance with your values, again and again, *is* the objective we're after in ACT. This is because if we become too goal focused, we can quickly fall into the trap of having the sense that we are OK only when we are achieving goals. For this reason, it is important to hold one's goals lightly and to use them as tools to valued living.

When articulating goals, it can be useful to generate SMART goals. SMART is an acronym that stands for **S**pecific, **M**easurable, **A**ction oriented, **R**ealistic, and within a specified **T**ime frame. For example, take the goal of "exercising more." What does "exercising" mean? Cardiovascular exercise or weight training? What does "more" mean, and over what time period will the exercise activity occur? The upcoming week? Each week? The upcoming year? How long will each period of exercise activity last? Thirty minutes? An hour? How will you know whether you've accomplished the goal of exercising more? As loose as the original formulation of "exercising more" is, it's at least action oriented—that is, it specified what will be done, not what won't be done. It did not read "be less sedentary." The goal will be realistic if it has a reasonable possibility of being accomplished, given the person's baseline. For example, if one has never run, it would not be realistic to set a goal of running 6 miles each day. However, if one has been averaging 6-mile runs each day, this would be more realistic, although perhaps not as growth oriented as it could be. The use of the SMART acronym increases the likelihood you will have addressed these important dimensions when you set your values-congruent goals.

Let's look at an example of Trent's goals (see pages 197–198). One of his values statements is "actively pursue hobbies and leisure activities." One of the goals tied to Trent's values is to practice performing "close-up" magic (e.g., advanced coin and card tricks performed within a few feet of the audience) three times each week, for at least 30 minutes per occasion over the next year. This goal is measurable, action oriented, and within a specified time frame. Practicing magic can include rehearsing routines, going over sleights, or reading new magic material in magic-related periodicals and books. All of this relates to the specific dimension on which Trent holds his focus for this practice. This is realistic given his current time commitments and given his baseline of one 30-minute period per week, with local club meeting attendance averaging every other month.

Below we provide an exercise to help you formulate your goals in a SMART format. Of course, you might wish to choose goals that relate to the problem area you have chosen for your ACT SP/SR work.

✍🏻 EXERCISE. My SMART Goals Worksheet

Chosen valued direction (the valued direction your SMART goals are to be related to):

_____

_____

_____

1. **Specific.** Articulate your goal with as much specificity as possible.

_____

_____

_____

2. **Measurable.** State your goal in a way that it can be measured effectively. Also decide how you will measure your progress toward your goal. Specify your goal in measurable terms here.

_____

_____

_____

3. **Action.** State your goals in terms of your behavior—that is, specify what it is that you will do. Use this question as a useful guide: "What would other people see me doing if I were achieving my goal?" List the specific behaviors they would observe here.

_____

_____

_____

4. **Relevant.** Reflect on whether your goals are directly related to your valued directions. If you achieved these goals, would that indicate you are living out your expressed values?

_____

_____

_____

5. **Time frame.** When do you plan to achieve this goal? Be specific. Would it be useful to specify short- and long-term goals? At what point in time will it make sense for you to pause and reflect on whether the goals were achieved?

_____

_____

_____

Final articulation of goal. Summarize the final formulation of your goal here.

_____

_____

_____

We have one other suggestion regarding goal setting. One secret to building large, sustainable patterns of values-driven behavior is to make sure the discrete behaviors that make up these larger patterns are reinforcing. When first developing valued patterns of committed action, you'll want your behavior to access reinforcement frequently. The best way to do this is to start with small steps. It can even be a good idea to start at or slightly below your baseline and then gradually increase the behavioral requirements. For example, if Trent's baseline was one 30-minute period of magic practice per week, he might want to start with a goal of 30, or even 25 minutes of practice each week (slightly below baseline) to ensure his behavior contacts reinforcement. This helps build momentum. Of course, the ultimate goal is to relate these discrete behaviors to values so that they consistently contact this form of intrinsic reinforcement and, thus build a large pattern of effective living.

 EXAMPLE: Trent's SMART Goals Worksheet

Chosen valued direction (the valued direction your SMART goals are to be related to):

Actively pursue hobbies and leisure activities. To be a nurturing and present father.

1. **Specific.** Articulate your goal with as much specificity as possible.
   I will engage in my hobby of performing close-up magic several times each week through practice and attendance at magician functions.

2. **Measurable.** State your goal in a way that it can be measured effectively. Also decide how you will measure your progress toward your goal. Specify your goal in measurable terms here.

   In terms of practice, I plan to practice at least three times each week, for at least 45 minutes on each occasion. The local magic club meetings occur once per month and are 2 hours in duration. I can measure this by tracking in a diary each time I practice and attend a magic meeting. I will graphically plot this each month.

3. **Action.** State your goals in terms of your behavior—that is, specify what it is that you will do. Use this question as a useful guide: "What would other people see me doing if I were achieving my goal?" List the specific behaviors they would observe here.

   I will read magic publications and practice sleights and full magic routines. I will attend monthly magic club meetings and will perform at least one effect at each meeting.

4. **Relevant.** Reflect on whether your goals are directly related to your valued directions. If you achieved these goals, would that indicate you are living out your expressed values?

   Yes, this is very much relevant. Achieving these goals will indicate I'm moving in my valued directions related to my children and also my recreational pursuits.

5. **Time Frame.** When do you plan to achieve this goal? Be specific. Would it be useful to specify short- and long-term goals? At what point in time will it make sense for you to pause and reflect on whether the goals were achieved?

   I plan to achieve the practice goals within the next 2 weeks—however, this is a weekly goal that I plan to maintain over the long term. The monthly magic meeting is about 3 weeks away and I plan to make my first attendance then. I plan to evaluate my progress toward both goals in 6 months.

Final articulation of goal. Summarize the final formulation of your goal here.

I will practice magic alone or with my children three times each week for at least 45 minutes on each occasion. Practice can include going over sleights, routines, or reading magic publications. I will also attend the local magic club meetings each month for their full duration. I will initiate progress toward these goals immediately and plan to have the initial pattern down within 2 weeks. I will evaluate my progress toward these goals in 6 months.

Identification of Barriers

So far, you have specified valued directions, chosen a direction to focus on, taken a baseline measurement of your effectiveness in living in accordance with your values, and you've specified goals tied to those values. We have one final step in this module, and that is to identify barriers to your committed action. Identifying barriers is important because this allows a strategy for overcoming them to be formulated. This advantage is enhanced by classifying identified barriers into one of two categories, each of which requires a different strategy for successful negotiation.

The first type of barrier is an internal one. In brief, this type of barrier occurs when certain psychological events emerged that we experience as aversive. We often respond to them as if they were literal, physical barriers. Consequently, our response is to try and avoid or escape those private events. The other type of barrier involves external factors. There are many examples of this kind of barrier, including various kinds of skills deficits and real-world circumstances, such as poverty.

Imagine you were at one end of a hallway and your goal was to get to the other end. If there were a large desk that was as wide as the hallway, effectively blocking your path, you would problem solve ways around that actual physical barrier. This would be logical and effective. In contrast, what if your destination goal was "blocked" by anxiety? Anxiety is not a physical object that must be physically negotiated, but nonetheless you might relate to this anxiety as if it were not much different from the desk. As you'll see in the next module, we make use of the barriers you identify here, as well as their differing classifications.

Examine the goals tied to the valued direction that is your current focus and list any barriers to executing your goals that you can identify. Use the form below to guide you in this process. For each barrier you identify, specify which type of barrier it is.

✍️ EXERCISE. My Barriers Identification

Write the values statement of concern and the SMART goal associated with it in the spaces provided below. Next, record the barriers connected to the SMART goal by writing them in the appropriate categories of internal and external.

Valued direction:

SMART goal linked to valued direction:

Barriers linked to execution of SMART goal:
Internal:

External:

Possible responses to barriers:

 EXAMPLE: Dennis's Barriers Identification

Valued direction:

Balancing completion of writing projects with spending time with family and loved ones. Establishing work/life balance while realizing vision for professional accomplishment and contributing to the scientific discussion and contributing to knowledge development.

SMART goal linked to valued direction:

Establishing a regular writing and project management schedule for Saturdays through Mondays. Waking before 6:00, and making time for meditation and writing before the flow of the day and family responsibilities begin.

Barriers linked to execution of SMART goal:

Internal:

Feeling tired and "overwhelmed" after a busy work week. Reluctance to wake early and begin when feeling overworked and tired. Feeling confused about where to begin on the weekend. Feeling "deprived" and craving engagement with entertainment and "relaxation," rather than work on a weekend morning. Anxious and self-critical thoughts when not engaging in work.

External:

Time demands from specific family gatherings and responsibilities. Limits of needed sleep. Need to engage in specific errands and housework. Time spent working on workshops and training that conflicts with this schedule. Backlog of administrative, billing, and email tasks that disrupts this schedule.

Possible responses to barriers:

Maintaining sleep/wake hygiene throughout the week. Integrating weekend scheduling with a larger schedule for the week to prevent intrusion of other tasks. Prioritizing early-morning project time over other arising tasks. Mindfulness, self-compassion, and defusion methods to respond to self-critical, anxiety-provoking, and permission-giving thoughts that can distract or interrupt the flow of work and enjoyment of time with family.

Self-Reflective Questions

What general observations do you have after completing the exercises in this module?

_____

_____

_____

_____

_____

_____

_____

_____

_____

_____

_____

Did you notice any thoughts, emotions, memories, bodily sensations, urges, or other private experiences that were particularly difficult for you to be willing to have? If so, were any of these new experiences or have they been traveling with you for a while?

_____

_____

_____

_____

_____

_____

_____

_____

_____

_____

_____

_____

_____

Which ways were most effective for you in opening up to and behaving through difficult private experiences?

_____

_____

_____

_____

_____

_____

_____

_____

_____

_____

_____

_____

Can you articulate at least one thing you might do differently with a client as a result of your experience with valued aims and SMART goals?

_____

_____

_____

_____

_____

_____

_____

_____

_____

_____

_____

_____

MODULE 12

Commitment, Part II
Cultivating Our Ability to Engage

In Module 10, you worked to identify important life directions. Once you articulated values statements, you generated SMART goals and identified barriers to their execution in Module 11. In this module, you'll work to execute these goals and to negotiate the identified barriers—that is, you'll work to engage in committed action.

Committed action is where living life happens. By way of analogy, imagine you were interested in learning to play golf, having never picked up a club before. There are many different component skills you must learn and master, such as the differing body mechanics for swinging a driver and putting with a putter. Once you acquire those component repertoires, you must then recruit them into the composite behavior we call "playing golf." Until now you've been working on the acquisition of several component repertoires, such as those involving defusion and present-moment awareness skills. Having now acquired these proficiencies, you are in a position to recruit these components into the composite behavior called "living life."

We begin your journey with committed action by helping you become acquainted with willingness.

Negotiating Internal Barriers: Building Your Capacity for Willingness

As we have seen together, willingness is an important capability to develop for effective living because it affords the key to negotiating painful internal content. Willingness is a difficult capability to describe because it can only be fully known through experiential practice. For example, Have you ever played a sport, or learned to play a musical instrument? For the sake of an example, let's continue with our golf discussion. Again, imagine you want to learn to play golf, and that you first want to learn the proper body mechanics for swinging a club. You could consult a golf instructor, who could describe those body mechanics in tremendous detail. You could also watch that instructor, and other golfers, swing. You could read extensively about the body mechanics involved. All of these activities would be helpful in your learning the proper body mechanics, but they would contain an important ceiling you could not surpass—that is, these methods would allow you to progress only so far. Why? Because the activity of swinging golf clubs involves nonverbal knowledge and thus can only be fully acquired through many experiences of club swinging. Willingness is very much like swinging a golf club in that it involves nonverbal knowledge.

EXERCISE. Intentional Discomfort: Meeting Willingness and Making It a Lifestyle

This is a very old practice, which involves building the psychic muscle that is necessary to establish and maintain commitment to our goals and valued aims. Over a century ago, the Armenian mystic and teacher George Gurdjieff described this process as intentional suffering—a deliberate and mindful engagement with discomfort in the service of pursuing our values (Lipsey, 2019). We aren't interested in contributing to suffering, but we are dedicated to building our capacity to accept discomfort and challenges with deep, mindful intention. So, in this exercise of "intentional discomfort," we build our ability to accept and expand our awareness around experiences that can pull us away from valued action.

Let's look at the process of dieting to explore the dynamics of commitment and engagement with discomfort. When we diet, we typically embark on an acute period of calorie restriction and increased exercise. This pattern is maintained until a goal weight is reached. However, the successful dieter does not then fully return to the predieting pattern of caloric consumption and activity. Instead, they adopt a new lifestyle pattern, the absence of which would surely result in regaining the weight they worked so hard to lose. The work we're asking you to do is very much like dieting. Initially, you will embark on an acute, intense pattern of behavior change, and to continue living the life you want, you'll need to make some permanent lifestyle changes. Those changes need not happen sequentially (i.e., behavior change followed by lifestyle change)—rather, they can occur simultaneously, as you are learning willingness experientially.

For this exercise we'd like you to identify and list some things you find irritating, but only moderately so. Next, we ask you to approach these things physically *and* psychologically, and to remain in their presence for a predetermined period of time. For this exercise to be useful, approaching these items should elicit private experiences you find uncomfortable. A moderate level of discomfort is ideal because discomfort that is too low will not afford a useful practice opportunity. In contrast, if the distress is too high, the experience may exceed your current capabilities, frustrating optimal learning. Importantly, we are not suggesting that you avoid items that produce a high magnitude of distress because doing so is dangerous. Indeed, this exercise is not dangerous. We are merely concerned with learning conditions.

Once you've identified items you find moderating distressing, the next step is to articulate how you will approach them in a SMART goal format. Next, you will make a commitment to stay in their presence for a specified period of time (e.g., 30 seconds, 1 minute, 10 minutes). It's important that you stipulate the length of time you will remain with the noxious item, before you execute the exercise. During the committed time periods, you are to solely practice noticing and allowing your thoughts, emotions, memories, bodily sensations, and the like to come and go—that is, you are to "just sit" with what shows up for you without any sort of white-knuckling or fighting with those experiences. You are to just let the experiences be.

Before we walk you through this exercise step-by-step, here are some examples of minor irritants:

- Listening to a type of music or artist you don't like.
- Hearing someone humming or whistling.
- Sitting in the presence of a food you really enjoy, and refraining from eating it.
- Listening to ambulance or fire sirens.
- Driving in heavy traffic or among discourteous drivers.
- Taking a cold shower.
- Surfing on a slow Internet.
- Engaging in a conversation with someone who goes "on and on."

There are two ways to approach this exercise. The first is with specific experiences that you can plan and initiate. For example, you can control whether you listen to annoying music by turning off such music at your convenience. The second approach involves taking advantage of these experiences when they occur naturally. An example is if you fine a particular person's whistling irritating, say a coworker, and you know you are likely to be in this person's presence while they whistle during the work week, you might commit to staying in your coworker's presence for 5 minutes or until they leave the situation. You can't control when and for how long your coworker shows up or how long they whistle, but you can control how long you will remain in their presence when they do so. Both approaches are useful. Importantly, *we are not suggesting at all that you should remain in the presence of any experience or situation that can cause you harm or injury. We don't advocate masochism or risk. So, holding a hot coffee cup, or walking through a highly trafficked area are definitely off of the list. This is an exercise in cultivating willingness to remain with discomfort, and not an exercise in punishment or risk taking.*

First, list routine minor irritants that you can produce or that are likely to happen naturally, here.

Specify how you will approach them here. Remember to use the SMART format to do so, to strive to do this at least once each day, and to specify how long you will commit to remaining in their presence.

Remember to take advantage of irritants when they occur naturally in addition to these scheduled practices. After 1 week of daily practice of willingly sitting with irritating experiences, provide your reflections on what you've learned from this exercise here.

Consider continuing this exercise for several more weeks. You might want to continue this daily, or you might want to experiment with alternating between willing and unwilling days, and then reflect on that experience. What's important is to begin developing a lifestyle characterized by willingness.

Commitment

Willingness and commitment go hand in hand. Willingness facilitates commitment, and commitment occasions the need for willingness. It is impossible to live life without experiencing thoughts, emotions, memories, bodily sensations, and so forth, many of which are painful. Living life and experiencing painful private experiences are not separable—they are one and the same. Consider the sport of boxing. There's no such thing as a boxer not getting hit. The only way for a boxer to not get punched is to refrain from boxing. Somewhat analogously, the only way to not experience painful private events is to not engage life.

Other important qualities of commitment exist. First, commitment is dichotomous. Either one commits or does not commit. There is no such thing as a "half" commitment. In the preceding exercise, you either committed to staying in the presence of an irritant for a specified period of time (e.g., 20 seconds, 1 minute), or you did not. This is an important quality and is the reason we asked you to commit to a specified duration before approaching the stimulus. Second, commitments can be titrated on various dimensions of magnitude only (e.g., time, frequency). You could have committed to a longer or a shorter time duration, and you could have selected a greater or lesser distressing stimulus to approach. However, you could not have chosen to alter your level of commitment once you were in the midst of the activity. You only could have chosen to escape the confronted stimulus. Finally, commitment does not require the provision of a guaranteed outcome. No one is capable of such an attestation. Rather, making a commitment means one is willing to invest in a course of behavior, and that if one is knocked off course, one will continuously reorient themselves to that trajectory.

ACT-Based Exposure

If it's not in your behavior, then it's not in your life. In the end, what matters is what you do. But when you start doing what's important to you, inevitably painful emotional barriers arise. Therefore, you must practice committing to a course of action that is tied to your values, and you must practice negotiating the private experiences that arise as a result. The most effective way for you to develop this expertise is for you to expose yourself to the contexts where you will need the new behavioral pattern and to practice emitting that pattern. Consider learning to swim. You could receive verbal instruction in swimming and you can read about it extensively. You could even spend time wading in the shallow end of a pool. But unless you have a substantial amount of experience swimming, in the locations and ways you will need to swim in the future, you will not become a strong swimmer. This next exercise provides a blueprint for practice of this kind.

EXERCISE. Exposure

This exercise of exposure involves getting to the heart of ACT SP/SR. This exercise will assist you in approaching important life contexts and recruiting your ACT competencies to those contexts so that you begin living more effectively. You can download an audio version of this practice from the book's website (see the box at the end of the table of contents), or alternatively, you can record the following script, perhaps into an appropriate app on your smartphone, and then listen to the recording to execute the exercise. When participating in the exercise, you have only to listen to, and follow, the instructions.

Gently close your eyes as you get comfortable where you are sitting. All you have to do during this exercise is listen to the sound of this voice.

First, let's get present. Begin by watching your breath—that is, watch the path that the air takes as you breathe in and out. Just watch as it travels up through your nose, down into your lungs, and in and out of your belly. When your mind wanders, as it will surely do, simply notice that it has wandered and gently bring it back to watching your breath. In fact, your only responsibility in this whole world is to simply watch your breath, here and now, so if it wanders 100 times, your job is to gently notice this and bring it back 100 times.

Once you feel a little more present, bring to mind an important goal tied to one of your valued directions. Perhaps this is a valued direction that is intimately tied to the problem you have chosen for this workbook. Importantly, recall a valued aim that is challenging for you to execute. The idea is to bring one to mind that will stir up difficult private experiences for you. Take the time you need for this process to unfold.

Once you have an important but challenging aim in mind, notice everything that is there to notice. Check in with each one of your senses. See what's there to be seen. Hear any sounds that are there to be heard. Get in touch with this experience as fully as you can, and do so as if you are there right now, not like you are watching this on a video screen. Observing yourself engaging with this valued aim. Notice where your mind goes as you watch yourself struggling with the challenge in the past. Imagine yourself facing the obstacles to this goal in the future. Allow any mental events that arrive with this valued aim to arise and move through your mind.

Follow wherever your engagement with this valued aim takes you, as deeply and closely as you can, moment by moment.

Take your time. Rest in the breath, and hold yourself in the presence of this very moment. Contact this experience vividly.

Once the experience is here and fully present for you, just sit still with the experience. Don't try to run from it or push it away. Rest in stillness, slowing your body and slowing your mind, and allow this experience to be there fully and without any defense. Just observe this experience.

Now, gently move your attention to your body. Notice all of the places in your body where this experience shows up. Just notice. We aren't running from or fighting with these bodily sensations. If you catch yourself fighting with them in any way, notice that you are doing so, and drop the struggle as much as you can, returning to simply noticing. Fully allow yourself to experience these bodily sensations.

Experience, as much as you can, what the experience of willingness of these bodily sensations is like. Can you notice this? If you had to rate, in your mind, how open you are, in this moment, to allowing yourself to experience these bodily sensations, from 0 to 10, how would you rate it? Regardless of how you rate your willingness, see whether you can sit with this long enough to increase your rating by at least 1. If you already rate it as a 10, see whether you can continue to sit in this space and observe what it's like to be willing at a 10.

Once you are more willing to allow those bodily sensations to be there, gently move your attention back to the original image—the one of you engaging with the pursuit of your valued aim. Get back in touch with all that's there to be seen, heard, and felt. Again, do this as if you are there now, not as though you are watching this on television. Allow that experience to come back fully.

When you are once again fully present to this experience, gently migrate your attention to any emotions that are present. Allow yourself to experience these emotional reactions fully. Let your attention give preference to absorbing the painful ones, if there are any. Just sit and notice these emotional reactions. Work to make room for these emotions and to allow yourself to experience them fully and without defense. These emotions are a part of your remembered history, and you need not fight with your history. See whether you can notice what it's like to become increasingly willing with your emotions. What's your willingness rating now? See whether you can continue to sit in this space until your willingness increases by at least 1. If your rating is already a 10, sit with this experience a bit longer while observing what it's like to feel willing at a 10 with your emotions.

Now, once again bring your attention back to the image—again observing it in the first person. See whether you can approach it even more boldly than you did before, with a posture of willingness.

Approach it with open arms.

Once you are again in contact with this experience, allow your attention to move to your thoughts. Matter-of-factly notice what thoughts are there. Notice any images. Notice any judgments or evaluations. As you notice, simply allow what you observe to be there fully and without defense. Try not to push any of this away or attempt to distract yourself from it. Just sit with it. See whether you can even approach those you find most troubling and whether you can do so gently and with compassion. What is your willingness rating now? Can you increase your willingness by 1? If you are already at a 10, see whether you can notice the quality of being willing to sit with your thoughts at a 10.

Once again, return to the original image. Try to experience it fully.

Once that experience is back and present for you, what is your overall willingness rating?

Continue until you are able to be willing to have these bodily sensations, emotions, and thoughts at an 8 or higher.

Continue until you achieve this.

Debriefing the exercise with yourself, describe your general observations here.

Were there any private experiences that were particularly difficult for you to be willing to have? If so, list those here.

If you listed any difficult experiences above, what skills from previous modules could you use to loosen up their grip on you, such as defusion techniques? Can you incorporate this into your next exposure practice?

Practice this exercise daily for at least 1 week.

The "ACT Formula" for Living an Open, Centered, and Engaged Life

There's a useful acronym that succinctly summarizes our approach to committed action: "ACT." The elements of the acronym are **A**ccept what private experiences are present by approaching them willingly, **C**hoose a valued direction to orient toward in this moment, and **T**ake action by moving in that direction (Harris, 2009). Repeat continuously.

Below is a two-part exercise. In Part I, you look retrospectively at a time where you became inflexible and then practice specifying how you could have "ACT-ed" differently in that circumstance. In Part II, you practice "ACT-ing" prospectively.

 EXERCISE. Accept, Choose, and Take Action

PART I

Situation

Think of a specific time, the more recent the better, when you noticed a shift in your mood, got hooked by a thought, or felt substantially less vital. Preferably, this is a time that relates to the problem area you have chosen for our work. Once you have a specific instance in mind, record a basic description of it here.

Accept what's there to be accepted.

Now, list all of the private events (thoughts, emotions, bodily sensations, memories, etc.) that were there and were difficult to accept.

List how you could have increased your willingness to experience those private experiences.

Choose a direction.

Record an important valued direction that you could have oriented toward in that specific circumstance.

Take action in that direction.

Specifically describe how you could have behaved in that valued direction.

You may want to do this on another two to three situations to enhance your learning.

PART II

For each of the next 7 days, complete this on at least one circumstance where you notice a shift in your mood, get hooked by a painful thought, or otherwise feel constricted.

Situation

When you notice a shift in your mood, got hooked by a thought, or feel substantially less vital, use this as a cue to complete this exercise. Briefly describe the circumstance here.

Accept what is there to be accepted.

List all of the private events (thoughts, emotions, bodily sensations, memories, etc.) that are present and in need of acceptance.

Can you be willing to have these experiences? Can you let go of the struggle? List what skills you will use to increase your willingness to have these experiences.

Use these skills to increase your willingness, right now, in this moment. And then . . .

Choose a direction.

Record an important valued direction that you can orient toward right now. What do you want to be about in this moment?

Take action in that direction.

Specifically describe how you will behave in that valued direction right now in this moment.

Move in that direction now!

💭 Self-Reflective Questions

What was your experience of completing the exercises in this module?

_____

_____

_____

_____

_____

_____

_____

_____

_____

_____

Did you notice any thoughts, emotions, memories, bodily sensations, urges, or other private experiences that were particularly difficult for you to be willing to have? If so, were any of these new experiences or have they been traveling with you for a while?

_____

_____

_____

_____

_____

_____

_____

_____

_____

_____

_____

_____

Which ways were most effective for you in opening up to and behaving through difficult private experiences?

_____

_____

_____

_____

_____

_____

_____

_____

_____

_____

_____

_____

Can you articulate at least one thing you might do differently with a client as a result of your experience with committed action? What would this look like in your personal life? What would it look like in your work as a clinician?

_____

_____

_____

_____

_____

_____

_____

_____

_____

_____

_____

_____

What would be essential for your plan for maintaining a long-standing pattern of committed action as a person and as a clinician?

_____

_____

_____

_____

_____

_____

_____

_____

_____

_____

_____

_____

SECTION E

COMPASSIONATE

ACT and Compassion

Over the last several years, many ACT practitioners have come to regard compassion as a central process in cultivating psychological flexibility (Dahl et al., 2009; Hayes, 2008; Neff & Tirch, 2013; Tirch et al., 2014). For thousands of years, compassion has been understood as a sensitivity to the presence of suffering in others and in oneself, coupled with a motivation and commitment to prevent and alleviate this suffering (Gilbert, 2010). Throughout history, spiritual and contemplative traditions the world over have prescribed training the mind in compassion as a way to deal with destructive emotional responses. Today, neuroimaging research (Weng et al., 2013), psychotherapy outcome research (Desbordes & Negi, 2013; Jazaieri, Urry, & Gross, 2013; Leaviss & Uttley, 2015), and psychological process research (Braehler et al., 2013; Gilbert, 2011; Gilbert et al., 2012; Weng et al., 2013) have all suggested that bringing a focus on compassion to our therapy may enhance our effectiveness. Rather than simply being an idea or an aspiration, we can understand compassion as an embodied human motivational imperative that has emerged from the evolution of human caregiving repertoires (Gilbert, 2010). As such, compassion involves our ability to stabilize ourselves in the presence of fear, and to turn toward life's challenges with greater flexibility and presence (Tirch et al., 2014). In this way, we can target compassion as an active process variable in our ACT SP/SR work.

According to Hayes (2008), compassionate action may be the one valued aim that inherently emerges from the psychological flexibility model. Hayes and colleagues (2006) describe an ACT-consistent conceptualization of compassion as involving:

- Willingly experiencing difficult emotions.
- Mindfully observing our self-evaluative, distressing, and shaming thoughts without allowing them to dominate our behavior or our states of mind.
- Engaging more fully in our life's pursuits with self-kindness and self-validation.
- Flexibly shifting our perspective toward a broader, transcendent sense of self.

This formulation clearly highlights the relationship between compassion and the elements of psychological flexibility that we have been cultivating.

When humans cultivate secure attachment relationships and experience affiliative motivations and affects, our minds are organized in ways that allow us to experience greater response flexibility, social safeness, and courage in the face of challenges (Gilbert, 2010; Johnson, 2012). Through this ACT SP/SR program, we are aiming to create a healthy context that can allow and encourage the growth of our own compassion for ourselves and others, bringing ourselves into deliberate contact with one of our greatest human capacities. Drawing on elements of CFT (Gilbert, 2010), a "fellow-traveler" school of therapy in the world of CBS, we can augment our ACT SP/SR practice of mindfulness and acceptance by consciously activating our compassionate mind (Kolts et al., 2018; Tirch et al., 2014).

Mindfulness, Compassion, and Acceptance

In the exercise that follows, we deliberately practice mindfulness, acceptance of difficult emotions, and compassion. We use rhythmic breathing, imagery, and self-direction to both cultivate these ways of being and to explore the relationships among mindfulness, compassion, and acceptance (MCA).

For centuries, mindfulness and compassion have been viewed as highly related states of mind in Buddhist mental training (Germer, 2009). Mindful Self-Compassion (MSC) program cofounder Christopher Germer has gone so far as to describe mindfulness and compassion as "two wings of a bird." Indeed, the MSC program defines "self-compassion" as consisting of a blend of mindful awareness, self-kindness, and a sense of our common humanity (Neff & Germer, 2013). From this point of view, mindfulness itself makes up a large part of the experience of self-compassion. In the classical compassion definition, which has been adapted and used by CFT and compassion-focused ACT practitioners, the first step in awakening compassion involves a present-moment-focused sensitivity to the presence of suffering in self and others. Mindfulness can be viewed as the doorway to that conscious sensitivity.

According to CFT theory and compassion assessment research, acceptance and distress tolerance are core attributes of our compassionate mind (Gilbert et al., 2017). A mind that is organized by compassion appears readier to willingly turn toward, and remain open to, suffering, in the service of the right action. Similarly, acceptance is generally considered to be a central aspect of mindfulness, too. Some definitions of mindfulness place acceptance at the heart of the concept. According to Boorstein (2003, p. 8), "Mindfulness is the aware, balanced acceptance of the present moment. It isn't more complicated than that. It is opening to receive the present moment, pleasant or unpleasant, just as it is, without either clinging to it or rejecting it." So, when we are practicing these three ways of being, we are activating highly interrelated aspects of our human potential that can help us to respond to life's challenges and opportunities with greater psychological flexibility.

Practicing MCA

The following practice walks us through the unfolding processes of MCA. Since evidence-based therapies love to distill the names of our techniques into their initials, our ACT SP/SR team has dubbed this experiential practice *MCA training*. Some have suggested that this name was meant to honor the memory of a prominent 20th-century Buddhist practitioner and human rights advocate, the late Adam "MCA" Yauch, but that has never been confirmed.

This MCA practice is particularly well suited to self-reflection and group discussion. Despite how interconnected the experience of MCA can seem, this exercise aims for us to encounter each of these dimensions of the awakening mind directly as they unfold into one another. For example, our capacity for mindfulness can allow us to notice the arising of an emotion or thought in the present moment. When we are able to hold ourselves in kindness, with our mind organized by our evolved caregiving motives, we can experience bodily and emotional states that better prepare us to turn toward difficult experiences. From this place of mindful compassion, we are better prepared to choose willingness and acceptance, rather than descending into EA. When practicing self-reflection after this exercise, part of our aim is to discriminate the function and the quality of experience of these three important processes. We invite you to emphasize this in your self-reflection questions and answers. Following that, you might find that group discussion of these nuanced distinctions can be very helpful in learning to work with MCA with precision and care.

The following instructions can be recorded so that you might practice MCA as a guided meditation. You can also download an audio version of this practice from the book's website (see the box at the end of the table of contents), or alternatively, you can read and memorize the following as guidelines for silent practice.

Find a space where you can be alone with relative quiet for several minutes. In this space, using a meditation cushion or chair, adopt a posture where you feel supported, with a straight, even slightly concave curve to your back. Allow your eyes to close and begin to gather your attention, center yourself, and practice mindful breathing.

As you begin, take three mindful breaths and feel the release of tension with each exhalation. Pay particular attention to the fullness of each exhalation. As much as you can, adopt an open and curious orientation to the physical sensations that accompany each breath.

Stay with the practice of mindful breathing for as long as you need, perhaps allowing yourself a few minutes of calm abiding in a mindful state. Whenever your mind wanders away from your gentle focus on the breath, allow yourself a moment of mindfully noticing whatever arrives—just making space for whatever arises in the moment.

On the next natural inhalation, bring mindful attention to physical sensations that emerge throughout the body. You may even say the word noticing *in your mind. In this moment, we are bringing mindfulness to this moment. We are opening to the presence of life in the body, and casting the light of our mindful awareness to the presence of our emotions as they arrive in physical sensation.*

Allow your mind to turn toward the challenging edge of your experience. Are there difficult emotions that arise in this moment? Allow and notice them. Are there distracting and challenging thoughts that move through your mind? Allow and notice them. Gently, gradually, the soft focus of our mindful attention shifts from the breath to our experience itself. We are mindfully aware of all that arrives in this moment—thoughts, emotions, and physical sensations.

Whatever arrives, allowing yourself to rest in the breath, feeling the movement of the abdomen and rib cage, bringing open, mindful attention to sensations in the heart center. Repeat the word noticing *in your mind. In this moment, bringing bare attention to the quality of your experience. Letting go of judgment. Noticing. Noticing.*

Mindful.

Mindful.

In this moment, present to whatever arrives, bringing compassion to physical experience through the breath. With this inhalation, we can feel compassionate attention moving toward our difficult thoughts and emotions.

With each exhalation, let go of unnecessary tension, bringing compassion to every experience of emotion throughout the body.

Whatever your emotional experience is, allowing yourself to feel it fully as physical sensation, while bringing great care and kindness to every breath.

Remember a time when you were in the presence of someone you cared for deeply. Recall looking into the eyes of this person who you would protect and love unconditionally. If no person comes to mind, perhaps you can remember an animal you had a special connection with. If no animal comes to mind, perhaps you can even remember yourself as a child.

Look into the innocence and hope behind the eyes of the you who was there and then. Imagine that this being is feeling difficult emotions.

As you remember, looking deeply into the person's eyes and connecting with their heart, imagining what it would be like to feel their suffering. Remembering what it would be like to feel sensitive to the person's suffering, and allowing the experience of being moved to do something to help them.

Connect with and notice your arising compassion.

Invite mindfulness and compassion into this moment.

Repeat the words in your mind—mindful and compassionate—*noticing and* caring— mindful *and* compassionate.

Gently breathe your attention to the places in the body where your difficult emotions have arrived. Invite your body to soften and relax around these sensations. Willingly making compassionate space for your emotions. Expanding compassionate attention to your physical experience of emotion. Reminding yourself that whatever arises in your mind and body, it's OK to experience it.

Mindful and compassionate.

Whatever arises in your mind and body, it's OK to experience it.

In this moment, your mindfulness and compassion are an invitation for your body and mind to soften and accept your experience. Your compassionate mind has the wisdom, strength, and commitment that you need to accept the fullness of your experience. Whatever arrives, saying hello to your experience. Standing in the gate of our awareness, we invite the totality of this moment. We say yes to this moment and all that it contains.

Mindful, compassionate, and accepting—mindful, compassionate, and accepting— mindful, compassionate, and accepting.

Stay with this process of resting in a state of mindfulness, compassion, and acceptance for a few minutes. In this moment, bringing caring and attention to your experience. If you'd like, place your hands over your heart—feeling the warmth of your hand against your heart, bringing kindness and strength to your experience.

Acknowledge and expand around any distress or struggle that arrives in this moment. Bringing mindfulness, compassion, and acceptance into contact with our experience of this moment, we are expanding around the vastness of our entire being.

Breathing in, we notice that we are breathing in, and breathing out, we notice that we are breathing out.

Forming an intention to let go of this practice, acknowledge the accomplishment and merit in moving toward greater mindfulness, compassion, and acceptance. In this moment, we offer up whatever merit we have gained in this practice to the liberation of suffering for all beings. May all beings be liberated from struggle and needless suffering. May all beings know meaning, purpose, and vitality. May we all know mindfulness, compassion, and acceptance. After a few mindful breaths, with a long cleansing exhalation, let this entire practice go.

The experiential exercise above can be used in a number of ways:

- It can be used to introduce and illustrate how MCA can flow into one another.
- It can be used to experientially learn how mindfulness can serve as a context for compassion, and how compassion can create an atmosphere of care and safeness that facilitates acceptance.
- It can be used as a daily meditation for practicing and cultivating MCA.
- The steps of moving from mindfulness to compassion and acceptance can be adapted as an in-the-moment tool that can help us to move toward psychological flexibility in the moment as we face life's challenges.
- In an applied and in vivo form, the entire exercise can be shortened to a few mindful breaths, evoking MCA through imagery, breath, and internally repeating "mindfulness, compassion, and acceptance."

An ACT SP/SR group can determine how they would like to implement this practice over the course of working through this module, and can share their observations through personal reflections or their notes from their regular meditative practice.

Self-Reflective Questions

What was your experience as you engaged in the MCA practice? What observations arrived during and just after your period of meditation? What did you learn about MCA?

_____

_____

_____

_____

_____

_____

_____

_____

_____

_____

_____

_____

What did you notice about how mindfulness, compassion, and acceptance relate to
one another? How are these concepts the same? How are they different? How did you
understand the experience of MCA?

_____

_____

_____

_____

_____

_____

_____

_____

_____

_____

From your experience, what would it be like to consciously bring MCA into your acceptance during a psychotherapy session? When else might it be useful to bring these qualities into contact with your experience?

_____

_____

_____

From your experience, how does psychological flexibility relate to the experience of intentionally focusing on MCA? Can we be accepting and committed to valued action while we hold a compassionate intention to alleviate and prevent suffering? Can we truly be accepting of our difficult experiences and the difficult experiences of others without a compassionate intention?

MODULE 14

Compassion and Empathic Distress Fatigue

As an ACT therapist, you are making a choice to be open to your clients' experience of human suffering in the service of helping them lead lives of meaning, purpose, and vitality. Necessarily, this means that you, yourself, will have frequent experiences of distressing thoughts and emotions. Just as a firefighter is more likely to feel extreme heat, you are more likely to face extreme emotions in your day-to-day, professional life. Understandably, exposing ourselves to emotional pain can lead to high levels of distress and burnout (Craig & Sprang, 2010; Figley, 2002). While ACT therapists are not more likely to experience problematic burnout levels than other therapists, some research with ACT trainees suggests that we might report higher levels of anxiety and emotional distress than CBT therapists doing similar work (Lappalainen et al., 2007). Given our emphasis on the full experience of our emotional lives, it is not surprising that we will come into conscious contact with challenging feeling states often. It is essential that we understand the dynamics of how our clients' pain can pain us, and how we can respond to our own distress, in the moment and effectively, in order to enhance our own psychological flexibility and avoid common clinical mistakes (Brock et al., 2015).

In popular psychology discussions, the term *compassion fatigue* is often used to describe how caregivers and clinicians may eventually become drained and depleted by their work. The term suggests that we draw upon an exhaustible reservoir of compassionate care, and that we eventually just run out of these resources. Recent research suggests that this isn't the case. Klimecki and Singer (2012) have suggested that *empathic distress fatigue* would be a better description of what occurs when clinicians begin to burn out and lose access to compassionate responding. When we deeply listen and observe the suffering of others, our body and brain respond in ways that are similar to the person who is suffering before us. For example, research suggests that an empathic observer will have the same brain regions stimulated as those active in a person who is sharing their experience of emotional pain (Singer, 2006; Singer & Frith, 2005; Singer, Kiebel, Winston, Dolan, & Frith, 2004; Singer, Seymour, et al., 2004). ACT therapists can understand this through the processes of flexible perspective taking and cognitive fusion. When I imagine and symbolically represent your pain, my own pain is evoked and experienced. In time, repeated and unbuffered exposure to empathic distress can have deleterious effects on us.

Importantly, the gradual buildup of stress that occurs from excessive empathic exposure to suffering has nothing to do with a decrease in our levels of compassion. In fact, our embodied experience of compassion involves our ability to mindfully remain in the presence of distress, while feeling stabilized and supported. Far from causing fatigue, activating our experience of self-compassion while we are exposed to empathic distress can help us to better deal with our own emotional pain. Supported by a conscious experience of self-compassion, we might be better able to respond to empathic distress fatigue. This means that we can remain more available to our patients, and can take better care of ourselves.

Compassion Circulation

The following exercise involves a practice of mindfully circulating a compassionate intention between you and another person. We use mindful breathing, brief self-statements, and imagination to establish a state of mind that might be more conducive to dealing with empathic distress fatigue as it arises. For the first week of practice, this exercise is best used like a typical, seated mindfulness practice. Set aside some time in a quiet place, on your own, to engage in this practice for about 5–10 minutes. We have provided an accompanying practice record on page 230 so that you might write down your observations about practicing circular compassion during your initial practice period.

The meditation itself is a modified form of Tonglen visualization, which traditionally involves breathing in the suffering of all beings and imagining compassion flowing out from you to all beings as you breathe out (Sogyal, 2012). In Japanese Vajrayana meditations, practitioners imagine breathing in the breath of the Buddha of compassion, and breathing out their own compassionate intention, which is received by a cosmic, compassionate Buddha (Chodron, 2001; Tirch et al., 2015; Young, 2016). In compassion-focused ACT (Tirch et al., 2014), CFT (Gilbert, 2010), and the MSC program (Neff & Germer, 2013), similar practices are used to stimulate an experience of a flow of compassion from ourself to others, and from others back to ourself. Rather than avoiding our experience of distress and threat-based processing, we aim to evoke the benefits of operating from a compassionate and flexible mode of mind, as we engage with suffering directly.

After you have practiced this meditation for a few days or weeks, you may wish to silently begin to bring the words of the exercise to mind during your clinical day. Imagine yourself sitting with a client when you begin to feel an increase in your distress. As this occurs, you mindfully make space for the physical sensations, emotions, and thoughts that are arising moment by moment. Rather than turning away from your experience, losing yourself in distraction, or shifting into an obsessive problem-solving mode, you can choose to bring a compassionate intention to your work, remaining empathically engaged without excessively activating your stress response in the process. You can download an audio version of this practice from the book's website (see the box at the end of the table of contents), or record yourself reading the instructions and play them back.

✍ EXERCISE. Compassion Circulation

As you begin, find a comfortable place to sit and allow your eyes to close. Breathing out, imagine yourself releasing any needless tension or defense.

Feeling the experience of release on the outbreath, allow a full exhalation.

Breathing in, notice the sensations of your inbreath. Feel the movement of the abdomen, breathing attention into the body.

Taking this time outside of "clock time," allow each breath to lengthen and extend. Practicing mindful awareness, allow your mind to simply rest in this present moment. As much as you can, adopting an attitude of open, accepting awareness, inviting a kind curiosity about what is here, now.

Whenever the mind wanders away from this present moment, simply notice and make space for that experience. While gently noticing the natural wanderings of awareness, bring your focus back to this very moment, noticing the physical sensations of this natural inbreath.

Breathing in, we know that we are breathing in. Breathing out, we know that we are breathing out. Remain with this mindful observation of the flow of your breathing for as long as is right for you, now.

When it feels right, with the next inbreath, imagine yourself saying the words "I am breathing in compassion for myself." Allow yourself to hear these words in your mind, and feel a flow of compassionate awareness in your body as you draw breath.

With the next oubreath, imagine yourself saying the words "I am breathing out compassion for you." As you breathe out, hear these words in your mind, and feel a physical flow of compassionate intention as you exhale.

You can imagine a client or person you know who is suffering when you practice this exercise on your own. If you are silently practicing this during a psychotherapy session, the person sitting across from you becomes the object of your outward flowing compassion.

Ground yourself in the physical experience of warmth, kindness, and compassion with each breath. Remain with this practice, circulating the breath of compassion between you and another person for a few minutes, and when you are ready to complete this practice, bring your attention back to the flow of your breath itself and gradually allow the words to fall away. When the time is right, release a long exhalation, open your eyes, and bring your attention back into the room and return your awareness to your day.

In order to bring the practice of circulating compassion more fully into your routine, you may wish to establish a regular time and place for practice, keeping a record of your experience and your observations. An example of a weekly practice record kept by one of us (Dennis) appears on the next page.

EXAMPLE: Dennis's Compassion Circulation Record

Date and Time	Duration	Observations
Mon., 5:30 pm	15 min	I felt a deep connection to my breathing and physical sensations that reminded me of my Zen practice. I felt less focused on the meaning of the compassion phrases.
Tues., 7:20 pm	10 min	Today, I was very aware of the reality of the suffering of my clients. Imagining their own suffering with compassion, while holding myself in kindness, felt encouraging.
Wed., 11:15 am	20 min	I was rushed today, and did this practice in my office after sitting in a lot of traffic. I felt uncomfortable in the chair at first. After some time, I felt strong sadness for one client and a deep care for both of us as we will face some traumatic material in session today.
Thurs., 6:30 pm	15 min	This felt routine today, and I was mostly focused on mindful breathing throughout.
Fri., 8:30 pm	15 min	I noticed the release of tension in my abdomen and throat in the outbreath during this practice period, in particular.
Sat.	n/a	I woke late, and needed to head off to do a number of errands. I didn't manage to return to the practice today. I am committed to continue.
Sun., 9:10 am	10 min	The practice felt light and nearly refreshing this morning. The quality of the light through the window was beautiful upon completion of the practice.

EXERCISE. My Compassion Circulation Record

Date and Time	Duration	Observations

Practice on the Cushion and in the Consultation Room

Like many of the ACT practices that are rooted in contemplative traditions, compassion circulation can be practiced as a "meditation," but the state of mind that is accessed through the experiential exercise is meant to become a part of everyday experience. With the encouragement of the ACT SP/SR group, we can begin to use a three-step process of division of attention and valued action to integrate compassion circulation into our work. The steps are as follows:

1. Grounded in the ACT therapeutic stance, we mindfully notice when we experience considerable distress when working with a client. This might show up as an intense physical feeling, a distraction, or an experience of being "hooked" or "fused" with the content being discussed.

2. Once we have mindfully noticed this moment of suffering, we can bring compassionate attention to our own experience and to the experience of our client. We begin to connect our breathing in with a conscious motivation to be compassionate to ourselves in this moment. We begin to connect our breathing out to directing compassionate attention to our client. This is done in the same way that we practice during the meditation above, and is meant to be a background to our experience rather than a distraction. We do this in the same way that a musician may count the beats of a piece of music, while still bringing full attention to the notes they are playing and their connection to the audience.

3. Grounded in our circulation of compassion, we mindfully return our attention in each present moment to the exchange that occurs between our clients and ourself. As ACT is an experiential therapy, our practice of self-compassion can give us the space and interior safeness we need to track the psychological flexibility processes that need attention in our clients' words and actions. Similarly, we might be better able to activate mindfulness, acceptance, and commitment processes within ourself when we are operating from a place of compassion and stability, rather than fusion with internalized threat-based perceptions.

Self-Reflective Questions

What was your experience as you engaged in the compassion circulation practice? What observations were most vivid to you in the moment? What did you learn?

_____

_____

_____

_____

_____

_____

_____

_____

_____

_____

_____

_____

How did you find practicing compassion circulation on a regular, structured basis? How were you able to integrate this practice into your daily routine?

_____

_____

_____

_____

_____

_____

_____

_____

_____

_____

From your experience, what would it be like to bring compassion circulation to mind in the flow of a psychotherapy session? When might it be useful to circulate compassion as a way to create space for acceptance of difficult experiences?

_____

_____

_____

_____

_____

_____

_____

_____

_____

_____

_____

From your experience, how do you think compassion circulation relates to the ACT model? How do you think practicing self-compassion and a flow of compassion outward might help foster psychological flexibility?

_____

_____

_____

_____

_____

_____

_____

_____

_____

_____

Maintaining and Enhancing the Cultivation of Psychological Flexibility

As we reach the completion of our ACT SP/SR journey together, we return to the central aim of ACT in practice: living lives of meaning, purpose, and vitality. We are reminded of the core dimensions of the psychological flexibility model, our ability to contact the present moment, as it is, and not as our mind tells us that it is; willingly letting go of unhelpful defenses, and deepening our perspective on what it means "to be," as we proceed to realize the ways of doing and being that embody the version of ourselves we most wish to manifest. This module allows us to review our ACT SP/SR process and to prepare to carry what we have learned further, maintaining and enhancing our psychological flexibility.

In this workbook, you chose a particular problem that had been challenging for you in your life. This may have been a problem that was showing up in your professional life, and it may have been a problem that was having an impact on your personal life, too. You have systematically applied the processes used in ACT to contact this problem, to develop a new relationship to the problem itself, and to build valued aims that will take you toward the life you wish to lead. Throughout the work, you have been addressing this problem as a part of the act of living a meaningful life, rather than as a way of getting rid of a distressing experience.

Our journey has walked us through what it means to be open, centered, and engaged. We have practiced cultivating MCA. Our perspective on our experiences has been explored, as we have examined what it means to live our values, committing to returning again in kindness to the path we have chosen, whenever we have strayed. We have also practiced circulating compassion for ourselves and for others, preparing our mind and body to engage with the suffering that we might encounter as we proceed in the course of our work as psychotherapists.

You may have engaged with this workbook alone, working with a colleague or supervisor, or as a part of a group experience of ACT SP/SR. If you have shared this work with a group, you may have shared some of your reflections along the way and discussed what it is like to experience ACT from the inside out, in a systematic and structured way. Even if you worked on your own, you have been guided through a series of self-reflection questions so that you might consolidate, integrate, and deepen your experience of this therapy. As you begin this final module, you can return to the self-reflection questions you have already answered, and briefly review some of the observations and reflections that you have written over the last weeks. When we complete a course of therapy, we may choose to take some time to reflect, journalize, and construct a course of habits and practices that can allow us to further our self-realization. Similarly, after an extended meditative retreat, or a course of study in a wisdom tradition, it can be useful to reflect upon our path thus far, and to set our mind to the road ahead. This module is meant to give you some space to do just that.

We also invite you to take some time to reflect upon your development as an ACT therapist as you complete this workbook. Take some time to think about what it has been like to experience the techniques and processes of ACT from the inside out. How has applying these processes directly to your own life differed from helping a client develop psychological flexibility through ACT? What have you noticed about the psychological flexibility model through ACT SP/SR that you had not noticed before? Are there ways that you had been stuck or inflexible that you had not noticed? Are there new strengths, or dimensions of your empowerment, that you just hadn't noticed that have emerged? As you complete your work, together with a colleague, or on your own, it can be deeply valuable to consider, reflect, and deepen our understanding of ACT by spending time with these questions.

EXERCISE. Revisiting Our Measures

We began our modules by using some measures of psychological flexibility and other mental experiences, in order to orient ourselves to the problem we were facing and our ACT work. Just as you did at the beginning of this workbook, complete the measures again, and score each measure below.

AAQ-II: POST-SP/SR

Below you will find a list of statements. Rate how true each statement is for you by circling a number next to it. Use the scale below to make your choice.

1	2	3	4	5	6	7
never true	very seldom true	seldom true	sometimes true	frequently true	almost always true	always true

1. My painful experiences and memories make it difficult for me to live a life that I would value.	1 2 3 4 5 6 7
2. I'm afraid of my feelings.	1 2 3 4 5 6 7
3. I worry about not being able to control my worries and feelings.	1 2 3 4 5 6 7
4. My painful memories prevent me from having a fulfilling life.	1 2 3 4 5 6 7

5. Emotions cause problems in my life.	1 2 3 4 5 6 7
6. It seems like most people are handling their lives better than I am.	1 2 3 4 5 6 7
7. Worries get in the way of my success.	1 2 3 4 5 6 7

From Bond et al. (2011). Reprinted with permission from Frank W. Bond in *Experiencing ACT from the Inside Out: A Self-Practice/Self-Reflection Workbook for Therapists* by Dennis Tirch, Laura R. Silberstein-Tirch, R. Trent Codd, III, Martin J. Brock, and M. Joann Wright (The Guilford Press, 2019). Purchasers of this book can download additional copies of this form (see the box at the end of the table of contents).

This is a one-factor measure of psychological inflexibility, or EA. Score the scale by summing the seven items. Higher scores equal greater levels of psychological inflexibility. The average (mean) score in a clinical population was 28.3 (*SD* 9.9), while in a nonclinical population it was 18.51 (*SD* 7.05). Scores of > 24–28 suggest probable current clinical distress and make future distress and functional impairment more likely (Bond et al., 2011).

Next, complete the PHQ-9 and GAD-7, and score and interpret them using the guidelines we provide on the next page.

PHQ-9: POST-SP/SR

Over the last 2 weeks, how often have you been bothered by the following problems?	Not at all	Several days	More than half the days	Nearly every day
1. Little interest or pleasure in doing things	0	1	2	3
2. Feeling down, depressed, or hopeless	0	1	2	3
3. Trouble falling or staying asleep, or sleeping too much	0	1	2	3
4. Feeling tired or having little energy	0	1	2	3
5. Poor appetite or overeating	0	1	2	3
6. Feeling bad about yourself—or that you are a failure or have let yourself or your family down	0	1	2	3
7. Trouble concentrating on things, such as reading the newspaper or watching television	0	1	2	3
8. Moving or speaking so slowly that other people could have noticed; or the opposite—being so fidgety or restless that you have been moving around a lot more than usual	0	1	2	3
9. Thoughts that you would be better off dead or of hurting yourself in some way	0	1	2	3

Copyright by Pfizer, Inc. Reprinted in *Experiencing ACT from the Inside Out: A Self-Practice/Self-Reflection Workbook for Therapists* by Dennis Tirch, Laura R. Silberstein-Tirch, R. Trent Codd, III, Martin J. Brock, and M. Joann Wright (The Guilford Press, 2019). This form is free to duplicate and use. Purchasers of this book can download additional copies of this form (see the box at the end of the table of contents).

After completing the above measure, simply sum your score. The table below explains how your score compares to how others with varying levels of depression and distress have scored.

0–4:	No indication of depression
5–9:	Indicative of mild depression
10–14:	Indicative of moderate depression
15–19:	Indicative of moderately severe depression
20–27:	Indicative of severe depression
	My score: _____

GAD-7: POST-SP/SR

Over the last 2 weeks, how often have you been bothered by the following problems?	Not at all	Several days	More than half the days	Nearly every day
1. Feeling nervous, anxious, or on edge	0	1	2	3
2. Not being able to stop or control worrying	0	1	2	3
3. Worrying too much about different things	0	1	2	3
4. Trouble relaxing	0	1	2	3
5. Being so restless that it is hard to sit still	0	1	2	3
6. Becoming easily annoyed or irritable	0	1	2	3
7. Feeling afraid as if something awful might happen	0	1	2	3

As you did with the previous measure, simply sum your score for the above items. The table below tells you how your score compares to others who have completed this same measure, with varying levels of anxiety present in their lives.

Scores of:	
0–4:	No indication of anxiety
5–9:	Indicative of mild anxiety
10–14:	Indicative of moderate anxiety
15–21:	Indicative of severe anxiety
	My score: _____

Just as we did at the beginning of this workbook, after completing these measures, we suggest that you reflect on your scores and what they might mean for you. If you find that you are in a clinically relevant or severe range of depression, anxiety, or psychological inflexibility, we highly suggest that you discuss this with a trusted professional. You might choose to reach out to a supervisor, therapist, mentor, or colleague. If you are in therapy, share this information with your therapist. If you do not have mental health support, we suggest that you exercise self-compassion and seek the help that you need. If you had a specific concern not assessed by these measures, and chose to use other measures, review those, complete them again, and score them, too.

At the beginning of this workbook, we suggested that you periodically use these assessment measures to see what has changed and grown during your ACT SP/SR work. If you opted to do this, you may wish to explore or graph your progress throughout this program. At a minimum, we invite you to compare your scores at the beginning of this program and at its completion. We are particularly interested in the cultivation of psychological flexibility as measured by the AAQ-II. Beyond just the scores, take some time to look at the individual items and see what has changed for you. Are there ways that you relate to your experience differently, now that you have practiced ACT from the inside out? What are your areas for growth? What patterns of responding and action still hook you, and how might you design a road forward that allows you to continuously cultivate MCA and committed action in this lifetime?

✍️ EXERCISE. Reflecting upon My Challenging Problem

Write the problem that you have worked with throughout this workbook below, as you formulated it earlier in the ACT SP/SR program.

MY CHALLENGING PROBLEM:

Now, reflecting upon your experience of the ACT SP/SR program, respond to the following questions.

As you complete your ACT SP/SR work, what do you notice that has changed about your response to this challenging problem (or other challenges in your life)?

Were there dimensions of psychological flexibility or specific techniques that you have found more helpful or powerful throughout this workbook? If so, which techniques were they, and what did you notice about these processes?

How will you support, develop, and strengthen your psychological flexibility throughout your life, moving forward? Are there specific practices to which you can commit as you strengthen and maintain your psychological flexibility?

What private events, such as unwanted thoughts and emotions, might be challenging as you continue to move toward realizing your valued aims?

What public behaviors, observable actions, and external events, such as avoidance-based behaviors and difficult environmental contexts, might be challenging as you continue to move toward living your values?

In addition to changes that relate directly to this challenge or problem, what other effects of your participation in the ACT SP/SR program have you noticed in your life?

EXERCISE. Reflecting upon Psychological Flexibility in My Professional Life

> How has your experience of ACT SP/SR from the inside out deepened or changed your understanding of your clients' experiences in ACT?
>
>
>
>
> Reflecting on your experience of the ACT SP/SR program, what have you learned that might be useful in your work with clients or in other aspects of your professional life?
>
>
>
>
> How might you bring the techniques and ACT processes that you have experienced in this workbook directly into the work that you do with clients?

Completion

All of us wish to thank you for engaging in this ACT SP/SR process. In a sense, we have all been taking part in this work together, even though we are separated by space and time. We have been in direct communication as we have deepened our practice together, experiencing ACT from the inside out. All of the examples we have used have been drawn from our actual lived experiences. Throughout the process of our own ACT SP/SR work, and the writing of this book, we have all deeply engaged with the process of cultivating psychological flexibility. We have sought to cultivate mindfulness, acceptance, and commitment, as much as we could in the years developing this program, as we walked through life's challenges, including losing family members, facing cancer, changing jobs, moving homes, and bringing new lives into the world. You have your own challenges and joys, and we all hope that the work we have shared can help you face the struggle and liberate yourself from needless suffering, as much as you can.

The ACT journey is a life's work, and it is nothing, if not a way to bring compassion, wisdom, and strength into contact with the inevitable suffering that we all face as a part of our human family. We wish every reader strength, support, and kindness as they move toward lives of meaning, purpose, and vitality. Our dear friend and mentor Kelly Wilson has said that people who can tolerate ambivalence can wade out into places that other people can never go. For us, this means that working on ourselves through ACT SP/SR can help us to access wholeness, resilience, courage, and love, as we deepen our experience of our work and ourselves. ACT and CBS involve a living community, and just as we wish you strength and grace on your journey, we hope that our community supports you on your path. Take good care of yourselves, friends. See you down the road.

Self-Reflective Questions

As you complete this ACT SP/SR work, how might you summarize or crystalize the experience in a few sentences? If you wish, write a "completion statement," or even a "completion poem" below.

_____

_____

_____

_____

_____

_____

_____

_____

_____

_____

_____

_____

_____

Upon reflection on your ACT SP/SR work as a whole, what do you find to be the most significant message for how you approach your personal life?

_____

_____

_____

_____

_____

_____

_____

_____

_____

_____

_____

Upon reflection on your ACT SP/SR work as a whole, what do you find to be the most significant message for how you approach your professional life?

_____

_____

_____

_____

_____

_____

_____

_____

_____

_____

_____

_____

Do you think it would be values consistent and/or worthwhile to continue using an ACT SP/SR approach in the future? How might you use ACT SP/SR with yourself, your colleagues, your trainees, or even your clients? What obstacles might get in the way, and how might you work with them?

_____

_____

_____

_____

_____

_____

_____

_____

_____

_____

_____

_____

References

Bach, P. A., & Moran, D. J. (2008). *ACT in practice: Case conceptualization in acceptance and commitment therapy.* Oakland, CA: New Harbinger.

Barnes-Holmes, D., Hayes, S. C., & Dymond, S. (2001). Self and self-directed rules. In S. C. Hayes, D. Barnes-Holmes, & B. Roche (Eds.), *Relational frame theory: A post-Skinnerian account of human language and cognition* (pp. 119–139). New York: Kluwer Academic/Plenum Press.

Batten, S. V. (2011). *Essentials of acceptance and commitment therapy.* London: SAGE.

Batten, S. V., & Santanello, A. P. (2009). A contextual behavioral approach to the role of emotion in psychotherapy supervision. *Training and Education in Professional Psychology, 3*(3), 148–156.

Beck, J. S. (2011). *Cognitive behavior therapy: Basics and beyond* (2nd ed.). New York: Guilford Press.

Bennett-Levy, J. (2019). Why therapists should walk the talk: The theoretical and empirical case for personal practice in therapist training and professional development. *Journal of Behavior Therapy and Experimental Psychiatry, 62,* 133–145.

Bennett-Levy, J., & Lee, N. K. (2014). Self-practice and self-reflection in cognitive behaviour therapy training: What factors influence trainees' engagement and experience of benefit? *Behavioural and Cognitive Psychotherapy, 42*(1), 48–64.

Bennett-Levy, J., Lee, N., Travers, K., Pohlman, S., & Hamernik, E. (2003). Cognitive therapy from the inside: Enhancing therapist skills through practising what we preach. *Behavioural and Cognitive Psychotherapy, 31*(2), 143–158.

Bennett-Levy, J., McManus, F., Westling, B. E., & Fennell, M. (2009). Acquiring and refining CBT skills and competencies: Which training methods are perceived to be most effective? *Behavioural and Cognitive Psychotherapy, 37*(5), 571–583.

Bennett-Levy, J., Thwaites, R., Haarhoff, B., & Perry, H. (2015). *Experiencing CBT from the inside out: A self-practice/self-reflection workbook for therapists.* New York: Guilford Press.

Bennett-Levy, J., Turner, F., Beaty, T., Smith, M., Paterson, B., & Farmer, S. (2001). The value of self-practice of cognitive therapy techniques and self-reflection in the training of cognitive therapists. *Behavioural and Cognitive Psychotherapy, 29*(2), 203–220.

Blackledge, J. T. (2007). Disrupting verbal processes: Cognitive defusion in acceptance and commitment therapy and other mindfulness-based psychotherapies. *The Psychological Record, 57,* 555–576.

Bonanno, G. A., Papa, A., Lalande, K., Westphal, M., & Coifman, K. (2004). The importance of being flexible: The ability to both enhance and suppress emotional expression predicts long-term adjustment. *Psychological Science, 15*(7), 482–487.

Bond, F. W., Hayes, S. C., Baer, R. A., Carpenter, K. M., Guenole, N., Orcutt, H. K., . . . Zettle, R. D. (2011). Preliminary psychometric properties of the Acceptance and Action Questionnaire–II: A revised measure of psychological inflexibility and experiential avoidance. *Behavior Therapy, 42*(4), 676–688.

Boorstein, S. (2011). *It's easier than you think: The Buddhist way to happiness.* New York: Harper-Collins.

Braehler, C., Gumley, A., Harper, J., Wallace, S., Norrie, J., & Gilbert, P. (2013). Exploring change processes in compassion focused therapy in psychosis: Results of a feasibility randomized controlled trial. *British Journal of Clinical Psychology, 52*(2), 199–214.

Brock, M. J., Batten, S. V., Walser, R. D., & Robb, H. B. (2015). Recognizing common clinical mistakes in ACT: A quick analysis and call to awareness. *Journal of Contextual Behavioral Science, 4*(3), 139–143.

Chodron, T. (2001). *Buddhism for beginners.* Boston: Shambhala.

Craig, C. D., & Sprang, G. (2010). Compassion satisfaction, compassion fatigue, and burnout in a national sample of trauma treatment therapists. *Anxiety, Stress, and Coping, 23*(3), 319–339.

Dahl, J. C., Plumb, J. C., Stewart, I., & Lundgren, T. (2009). *The art and science of valuing in psychotherapy: Helping clients discover, explore, and commit to valued action using acceptance and commitment therapy.* Oakland, CA: New Harbinger.

Dalai Lama. (2004). *Dzogchen: The heart essence of the great perfection.* Boulder, CO: Snow Lion.

Davis, M. L., Thwaites, R., Freeston, M. H., & Bennett-Levy, J. (2015). A measurable impact of a self-practice/self-reflection programme on the therapeutic skills of experienced cognitive-behavioural therapists. *Clinical Psychology and Psychotherapy, 22*(2), 176–184.

Deacon, T. W. (2011). *Incomplete nature: How mind emerged from matter.* New York: Norton.

Deikman, A. (1982). *The observing self: Mysticism and psychotherapy.* Boston: Beacon Press.

Desbordes, G., & Negi, L. T. (2013). A new era for mind studies: Training investigators in both scientific and contemplative methods of inquiry. *Frontiers in Human Neuroscience, 7,* 741.

Ellis, A. (1979). Is rational-emotive therapy stoical, humanistic, or spiritual? *Journal of Humanistic Psychology, 19*(3), 89–92.

Ellis, A., & Robb, H. (1994). Acceptance in rational-emotive therapy. In S. C. Hayes, N. S. Jacobson, V. M. Follette, & M. J. Dougher (Eds.), *Acceptance and change: Content and context in psychotherapy* (pp. 91–102). Oakland, CA: Context Press.

Farrand, P., Perry, J., & Linsley, S. (2010). Enhancing self-practice/self-reflection (SP/SR) approach to cognitive behaviour training through the use of reflective blogs. *Behavioural and Cognitive Psychotherapy, 38*(4), 473–477.

Farrell, J. M., & Shaw, I. A. (2018). *Experiencing schema therapy from the inside out: A self-practice/self-reflection workbook for therapists.* New York: Guilford Press.

Figley, C. R. (Ed.). (2002). *Treating compassion fatigue.* Abingdon, UK: Routledge.

Foody, M., Barnes-Holmes, Y., & Barnes-Holmes, D. (2012). The role of self in acceptance and commitment therapy. In L. McHugh, I. Stewart, & M. Williams (Eds.), *The self and perspective taking: Contributions and applications from modern behavioral science* (pp. 125–142). Oakland, CA: New Harbinger.

Foody, M., Barnes-Holmes, Y., Barnes-Holmes, D., Törneke, N., Luciano, C., Stewart, I., & McEnteggart, C. (2014). RFT for clinical use: The example of metaphor. *Journal of Contextual Behavioral Science, 3*(4), 305–313.

Gale, C., & Schröder, T. (2014). Experiences of self-practice/self-reflection in cognitive behavioural therapy: A meta-synthesis of qualitative studies. *Psychology and Psychotherapy: Theory, Research and Practice, 87*(4), 373–392.

Georgescu, S., & Brock, M. (2016). A contextual cognitive-behavioral therapy approach to clinical professional training: Inside the classroom. In J. Block-Lerner & L. Cardaciotto (Eds.), *The mindfulness-informed educator* (pp. 73–92). Abingdon, UK: Routledge.

Germer, C. K. (2009). *The mindful path to self-compassion: Freeing yourself from destructive thoughts and emotions.* New York: Guilford Press.

Gilbert, P. (2010). *Compassion focused therapy: Distinctive features*. Abingdon, UK: Routledge.

Gilbert, P. (2011). Shame in psychotherapy and the role of compassion focused therapy. In R. L. Dearing & J. P. Tangney (Eds.), *Shame in the therapy hour* (pp. 325–354). Washington, DC: American Psychological Association.

Gilbert, P., Catarino, F., Duarte, C., Matos, M., Kolts, R., Stubbs, J., . . . Basran, J. (2017). The development of compassionate engagement and action scales for self and others. *Journal of Compassionate Healthcare, 4,* 4.

Gilbert, P., McEwan, K., Gibbons, L., Chotai, S., Duarte, J., & Matos, M. (2012). Fears of compassion and happiness in relation to alexithymia, mindfulness, and self-criticism. *Psychology and Psychotherapy: Theory, Research and Practice, 85*(4), 374–390.

Golemen, D., & Davidson, R. (2017). *Altered traits.* New York: Penguin.

Harris, R. (2006). Embracing your demons: An overview of acceptance and commitment therapy. *Psychotherapy in Australia, 12*(4), 70–76.

Harris, R. (2009). *ACT made simple: An easy-to-read primer on acceptance and commitment therapy.* Oakland, CA: New Harbinger.

Hayes, A. M., & Feldman, G. (2004). Clarifying the construct of mindfulness in the context of emotion regulation and the process of change in therapy. *Clinical Psychology: Science and Practice, 11*(3), 255–262.

Hayes, L. L., & Ciarrochi, J. V. (2015). *The thriving adolescent: Using acceptance and commitment therapy and positive psychology to help teens manage emotions, achieve goals, and build connection.* Oakland, CA: New Harbinger.

Hayes, S. C. (1993). Analytic goals and the varieties of scientific contextualism. In S. C. Hayes, L. J. Hayes, H. W. Reese, & T. R. Sarbin (Eds.), *Varieties of scientific contextualism* (pp. 11–27). Reno, NV: Context Press.

Hayes, S. C. (2004). Acceptance and commitment therapy, relational frame theory, and the third wave of behavioral and cognitive therapies. *Behavior Therapy, 35*(4), 639–665.

Hayes, S. C. (2005). *Get out of your mind and into your life: The new acceptance and commitment therapy.* Oakland, CA: New Harbinger.

Hayes, S. C. (2008). *The roots of compassion.* Keynote address presented at the fourth Acceptance and Commitment Therapy Summer Institute, Chicago, IL.

Hayes, S. C. (2016, March). *Psychological flexibility: How love turns pain into purpose* (TEDx University of Nevada). Retrieved from *www.youtube.com/watch?v=o79_gmO5ppg.*

Hayes, S. C., Barnes-Holmes, D., & Roche, B. (Eds.). (2001). *Relational frame theory: A post-Skinnerian account of human language and cognition.* New York: Springer.

Hayes, S. C., & Lillis, J. (2012). *Acceptance and commitment therapy.* Washington, DC: American Psychological Association.

Hayes, S. C., & Long, D. (2013). Contextual behavioral science, evolution, and scientific epistemology. In B. Roche & S. Dymond (Eds.), *Advances in relational frame theory: Research and application* (pp. 5–26). Oakland, CA: New Harbinger/Context Press.

Hayes, S. C., Luoma, J. B., Bond, F. W., Masuda, A., & Lillis, J. (2006). Acceptance and commitment therapy: Model, processes and outcomes. *Behaviour Research and Therapy, 44*(1), 1–25.

Hayes, S. C., & Shenk, C. (2004). Operationalizing mindfulness without unnecessary attachments. *Clinical Psychology: Science and Practice, 11*(3), 249–254.

Hayes, S. C., Strosahl, K. D., & Wilson, K. G. (1999). *Acceptance and commitment therapy: An experiential approach to behavior change.* New York: Guilford Press.

Hayes, S. C., Strosahl, K. D., & Wilson, K. G. (2012). *Acceptance and commitment therapy: The process and practice of mindful change* (2nd ed.). New York: Guilford Press.

Hayes, S. C., Wilson, K. G., Gifford, E. V., Follette, V. M., & Strosahl, K. (1996). Experiential avoidance and behavioral disorders: A functional dimensional approach to diagnosis and treatment. *Journal of Consulting and Clinical Psychology, 64*(6), 1152–1168.

Hooper, N., & Larsson, A. (2015). *The research journey of acceptance and commitment therapy (ACT).* New York: Springer.

Hooper, N., Saunders, J., & McHugh, L. (2010). The derived generalization of thought suppression. *Learning and Behavior, 38*(2), 160–168.

Huppert, J. D., & Alley, A. C. (2004). The clinical application of emotion research in generalized anxiety disorder: Some proposed procedures. *Cognitive and Behavioral Practice, 11*(4), 387–392.

Jazaieri, H., Urry, H. L., & Gross, J. J. (2013). Affective disturbance and psychopathology: An emotion regulation perspective. *Journal of Experimental Psychopathology, 4*(5), 584–599.

Johnson, S. M. (2012). *The practice of emotionally focused couple therapy: Creating connection.* New York: Routledge.

Kabat-Zinn, J. (2013). *Full catastrophe living: How to cope with stress, pain and illness using mindfulness meditation* (rev. ed.). London: Hachette.

Kashdan, T. B., Barrios, V., Forsyth, J. P., & Steger, M. F. (2006). Experiential avoidance as a generalized psychological vulnerability: Comparisons with coping and emotion regulation strategies. *Behaviour Research and Therapy, 44*(9), 1301–1320.

Kashdan, T. B., & Rottenberg, J. (2010). Psychological flexibility as a fundamental aspect of health. *Clinical Psychology Review, 30*(7), 865–878.

Klimecki, O., & Singer, T. (2012). Empathic distress fatigue rather than compassion fatigue?: Integrating findings from empathy research in psychology and social neuroscience. In B. Oakley, A. Knafo, G. Madhavan, & D. S. Wilson (Eds.), *Pathological altruism* (pp. 368–383). New York: Oxford University Press.

Kolts, R. L., Bell, T., Bennett-Levy, J., & Irons, C. (2018). *Experiencing compassion-focused therapy from the inside out: A self-practice/self-reflection workbook for therapists.* New York: Guilford Press.

Kroenke, K., Spitzer, R. L., & Williams, J. B. (2001). The PHQ-9: Validity of a brief depression severity measure. *Journal of General Internal Medicine, 16*(9), 606–613.

Lappalainen, R., Lehtonen, T., Skarp, E., Taubert, E., Ojanen, M., & Hayes, S. C. (2007). The impact of CBT and ACT models using psychology trainee therapists: A preliminary controlled effectiveness trial. *Behavior Modification, 31,* 488–511.

Leahy, R. L. (2017). *Cognitive therapy techniques: A practitioner's guide* (2nd ed.). New York: Guilford Press.

Leaviss, J., & Uttley, L. (2015). Psychotherapeutic benefits of compassion-focused therapy: An early systematic review. *Psychological Medicine, 45*(5), 927–945.

Lipsey, R. (2019). *Gurdjieff reconsidered: The life, the teachings, the legacy.* Boulder, CO: Shambhala.

Luoma, J. B., Hayes, S. C., & Walser, R. D. (2007). *Learning ACT: An acceptance & commitment therapy skills-training manual for therapists.* Oakland, CA: New Harbinger.

Luoma, J. B., & Vilardaga, J. P. (2013). Improving therapist psychological flexibility while training acceptance and commitment therapy: A pilot study. *Cognitive Behaviour Therapy, 42*(1), 1–8.

Marcks, B. A., & Woods, D. W. (2005). A comparison of thought suppression to an acceptance-based technique in the management of personal intrusive thoughts: A controlled evaluation. *Behaviour Research and Therapy, 43*(4), 433–445.

Mathews, A. (1990). Why worry?: The cognitive function of anxiety. *Behaviour Research and Therapy, 28*(6), 455–468.

McHugh, L., Stewart, I., & Hooper, N. (2012) A contemporary functional analytic account of perspective taking. In L. McHugh, I. Stewart, & M. Williams (Eds.), *The self and perspective taking: Contributions and applications from modern behavioral science* (pp. 55–72). Oakland, CA: New Harbinger.

Moran, D. J., Bach, P., & Batten, S. (2018). *Committed action in practice.* Oakland, CA: New Harbinger.

Neff, K. D., & Germer, C. K. (2013). A pilot study and randomized controlled trial of the mindful self-compassion program. *Journal of Clinical Psychology, 69*(1), 28–44.

Neff, K., & Tirch, D. (2013). Self-compassion and ACT. In T. B. Kashdan & J. Ciarrochi (Eds.), *Mindfulness, acceptance, and positive psychology: The seven foundations of well-being* (pp. 78–106). Oakland, CA: Context Press/New Harbinger.

Norcross, J. C., & Lambert, M. J. (2011). Psychotherapy relationships that work II. *Psychotherapy, 48*(1), 4–8.

Pakenham, K. I. (2015). Effects of acceptance and commitment therapy (ACT) training on clinical psychology trainee stress, therapist skills and attributes, and ACT processes. *Clinical Psychology and Psychotherapy, 22*(6), 647–655.

Pakenham, K. I., & Stafford-Brown, J. (2012). Stress in clinical psychology trainees: Current research status and future directions. *Australian Psychologist, 47*(3), 147–155.

Polk, M. (2014). Achieving the promise of transdisciplinarity: A critical exploration of the relationship between transdisciplinary research and societal problem solving. *Sustainability Science, 9*(4), 439–451.

Polk, M. (2015). Transdisciplinary co-production: Designing and testing a transdisciplinary research framework for societal problem solving. *Futures, 65*, 110–122.

Powers, M. B., Zum Vorde Sive Vörding, M. B., & Emmelkamp, P. M. (2009). Acceptance and commitment therapy: A meta-analytic review. *Psychotherapy and Psychosomatics, 78*(2), 73–80.

Rogers, C. R. (1951). *Client-centered therapy: Its current practice, implications, and theory.* New York: Houghton Mifflin.

Rogers, C. R. (1957). The necessary and sufficient conditions of therapeutic personality change. *Journal of Consulting Psychology, 21*(2), 95–103.

Ruiz, F. J. (2010). A review of acceptance and commitment therapy (ACT) empirical evidence: Correlational, experimental psychopathology, component and outcome studies. *International Journal of Psychology and Psychological Therapy, 10*(1), 125–162.

Sanders, D., & Bennett-Levy, J. (2010). When therapists have problems: What can CBT do for us. In M. Mueller, H. Kennerley, F. McManus, & D. Westbrook (Eds.), *The Oxford guide to surviving as a CBT therapist* (pp. 457–480). Oxford, UK: Oxford University Press.

Schoendorff, B., Webster, M., & Polk, K. (2014). Under the hood: Basic processes underlying the matrix. In K. Polk & B. Schoendorff (Eds.), *The ACT matrix: A new approach to building psychological flexibility across settings and populations* (pp. 15–38). Oakland, CA: New Harbinger.

Schön, D. A. (1983). *The reflective practitioner: How professionals think in action.* New York: Basic Books.

Singer, T. (2006). The neuronal basis and ontogeny of empathy and mind reading: Review of literature and implications for future research. *Neuroscience and Biobehavioral Reviews, 30*(6), 855–863.

Singer, T., & Frith, C. (2005). The painful side of empathy. *Nature Neuroscience, 8*(7), 845–846.

Singer, T., Kiebel, S. J., Winston, J. S., Dolan, R. J., & Frith, C. D. (2004). Brain responses to the acquired moral status of faces. *Neuron, 41*(4), 653–662.

Singer, T., Seymour, B., O'Doherty, J., Kaube, H., Dolan, R. J., & Frith, C. D. (2004). Empathy for pain involves the affective but not sensory components of pain. *Science, 303*, 1157–1162.

Sogyal, R. (2012). *The Tibetan book of living and dying: A spiritual classic from one of the foremost interpreters of Tibetan Buddhism to the West.* New York: Random House.

Spendelow, J. S., & Butler, L. J. (2016). Reported positive and negative outcomes associated with a self-practice/self-reflection cognitive-behavioural therapy exercise for CBT trainees. *Psychotherapy Research, 26*(5), 602–611.

Spitzer, R. L., Kroenke, K., Williams, J. B., & Löwe, B. (2006). A brief measure for assessing generalized anxiety disorder: The GAD-7. *Archives of Internal Medicine, 166*(10), 1092–1097.

Stafford-Brown, J., & Pakenham, K. I. (2012). The effectiveness of an ACT informed intervention for managing stress and improving therapist qualities in clinical psychology trainees. *Journal of Clinical Psychology, 68*(6), 592–613.

Thwaites, R., Cairns, L., Bennett-Levy, J., Johnston, L., Lowrie, R., Robinson, A., & Perry, H. (2015).

Developing metacompetence in low intensity cognitive-behavioural therapy (CBT) interventions: Evaluating a self-practice/self-reflection programme for experienced low intensity CBT practitioners. *Australian Psychologist, 50*(5), 311–321.

Tirch, D., Schoendorff, B., & Silberstein, L. R. (2014). *The ACT practitioner's guide to the science of compassion: Tools for fostering psychological flexibility.* Oakland, CA: New Harbinger.

Tirch, D., Silberstein, L. R., & Kolts, R. L. (2015). *Buddhist psychology and cognitive-behavioral therapy: A clinician's guide.* New York: Guilford Press.

Titchener, E. B. (1916). *A text-book of psychology.* New York: Macmillan.

Tsai, M., Kohlenberg, R. J., Kanter, J. W., Holman, G. I., & Loudon, M. P. (2012). *Functional analytic psychotherapy: Distinctive features.* Abingdon, UK: Routledge.

Villatte, M., Villatte, J. L., & Hayes, S. C. (2015). *Mastering the clinical conversation: Language as intervention.* New York: Guilford Press.

Waller, G. (2009). Evidence-based treatment and therapist drift. *Behaviour Research and Therapy, 47*(2), 119–127.

Waller, G., Stringer, H., & Meyer, C. (2012). What cognitive behavioral techniques do therapists report using when delivering cognitive behavioral therapy for the eating disorders? *Journal of Consulting and Clinical Psychology, 80*(1), 171–175.

Walser, R. D., Karlin, B. E., Trockel, M., Mazina, B., & Taylor, C. B. (2013). Training in and implementation of acceptance and commitment therapy for depression in the Veterans Health Administration: Therapist and patient outcomes. *Behaviour Research and Therapy, 51*(9), 555–563.

Wegner, D. M. (1994). Ironic processes of mental control. *Psychological Review, 101*(1), 34–52.

Wegner, D. M., & Gold, D. B. (1995). Fanning old flames: Emotional and cognitive effects of suppressing thoughts of a past relationship. *Journal of Personality and Social Psychology, 68*(5), 782–792.

Wegner, D. M., Schneider, D. J., Knutson, B., & McMahon, S. R. (1991). Polluting the stream of consciousness: The effect of thought suppression on the mind's environment. *Cognitive Therapy and Research, 15*(2), 141–152.

Weng, H. Y., Fox, A. S., Shackman, A. J., Stodola, D. E., Caldwell, J. Z., Olson, M. C., . . . Davidson, R. J. (2013). Compassion training alters altruism and neural responses to suffering. *Psychological Science, 24*(7), 1171–1180.

Wenzlaff, R. M., & Wegner, D. M. (2000). Thought suppression. *Annual Review of Psychology, 51*(1), 59–91.

Westrup, B. (2014). Family-centered developmentally supportive care. *NeoReviews, 15*(8), e325–e335.

Wetterneck, C. T., Lee, E. B., Smith, A. H., & Hart, J. M. (2013). Courage, self-compassion, and values in obsessive-compulsive disorder. *Journal of Contextual Behavioral Science, 2*(3–4), 68–73.

Wilson, K. G., & DuFrene, T. (2009). *Mindfulness for two: An acceptance and commitment therapy approach to mindfulness in psychotherapy.* Oakland, CA: New Harbinger.

Wilson, K. G., & DuFrene, T. (2012). *The wisdom to know the difference.* Oakland, CA: New Harbinger.

Wilson, K. G., & Murrell, A. (2004). Values work in acceptance and commitment therapy: Setting a course for behavioral treatment. In S. C. Hayes, V. M. Follette, & M. M. Linehan (Eds.), *Mindfulness and acceptance: Expanding the cognitive-behavioral tradition* (pp. 120–151). New York: Guilford Press.

Yadavaia, J. E., Hayes, S. C., & Vilardaga, R. (2014). Using acceptance and commitment therapy to increase self-compassion: A randomized controlled trial. *Journal of Contextual Behavioral Science, 3*(4), 248–257.

Young, S. (2016). *The science of enlightenment: How meditation works.* Boulder, CO: Sounds True.

Yu, L., Norton, S., & McCracken, L. M. (2017). Change in "self-as-context" ("perspective-taking") occurs in acceptance and commitment therapy for people with chronic pain and is associated with improved functioning. *Journal of Pain, 18*(6), 664–672.

Index

Note. Page numbers in *italics* indicate a figure

251

Psychological flexibility (cont.)
  contacting the present moment, 72, 78, 79
  definition and concept of, 5–6, 78
  flexible perspective taking, 72, 136
  fusion and, 71
  as the goal of ACT SP/SR, 60
  maintaining and enhancing the cultivation of, 234–243
  present-moment awareness and, 118
  transcending attachment to self-stories, 63
  values authorship and, 181
  Kelly Wilson's description of, 104
Psychological flexibility model
  acceptance, 79–81
  committed action, 90–92
  contacting the present moment, 84–85
  defusion, 81–83
  overview of the hexaflex model, 78–79
  self-as-context, 85–87
  self-reflective questions, 92–95
  values authorship, 88–90
Psychotherapy
  development and growth of the SP/SR approach, 7
  perspective taking and, 137
Public events, in the ACT matrix, 98, 99
Public function-focused reflection, 50–51

Recall, strategies to aid, 41–42
Reflecting upon My Challenging Problem (exercise), 238–240
Reflection
  ACT therapeutic stance and reflection-in-action, 29–30
  engaging in the process of, 40–42
  individual differences in the capacities and motivations for, 39
  preparing for, 39–40
  public function-focused reflection, 50–51
Reinforcement, 197
Relational frame theory (RFT)
  clinical implications of, 18–19
  deictic framing, 136
  importance to ACT, 23, 26
  key concepts as clinical building blocks, 24–26
  overview and description of, 17–18
  self-reflective questions, 20–22
Resistance, to self-reflection, 39–40
Revisiting Our Measures (exercise), 235–238
RFT. See Relational frame theory

Safety, of participants in the ACT SP/SR program, 50–51
Schema therapy, 23
Self
  conceptualized self, 128–132
  senses of, 86
  separating thoughts from the thinker, 152–153
  transcendent self, 85
  See also Observer self
Self-as-content, 128–132
Self-as-context
  concept of, 85–86, 128
  "I Am . . ." exercise, 129
  The Ocean of Being exercise, 130–132
  psychological flexibility and, 78, 79
  self-as-content and, 128–132
  self-practice exercise, 86–7
  self-reflective questions, 133–135
Self-as-ongoing awareness, 86
Self-as-process, 86
Self-compassion, 41
Self-criticism, 130
Self-esteem, 130
Self-guided ACT SP/SR, 33
Self-practice and self-reflection (SP/SR) training
  application to other psychotherapies, 22–23
  building reflective capacity, 39–42
  development and growth of, 7–8
  overview, 3
  See also ACT SP/SR
Self-Practice Exercises
  with Acceptance, 80–81
  with Committed Action, 91–92
  with Contacting the Present Moment, 84–85
  with Defusion, 82–83
  with Self-as Context, 86–87
  with Values Authorship, 88–89
Self-reflection
  building reflective capacity, 39–42
  See also Reflection; Self-practice and self-reflection training
Self-reflective questions
  for acceptance and willingness, 172–175
  for the ACT matrix, 109–113
  for the ACT SP/SR challenge formulation, 75–77
  for committed action, 201–203, 213–215
  for compassion circulation, 231–233
  for the conclusion of the ACT SP/SR process, 241–243
  for contacting the present moment, 125–127
  for defusion, 154–157
  for flexible perspective taking, 142–144

for functional contextualism, 14–17
for identifying one's challenging problem, 67–69
for mindfulness, compassion, and acceptance, 223–225
for psychological flexibility, 92–95
for relational frame theory, 20–22
for self-as-context, 133–135
using to guide recall, 42
for values authorship, 187–190
Self-reflective writing, 42
Sensory experiencing, versus mental experiencing, 100–101
Shame, 130
SMART goals
  concept of, 195–196
  My Barriers Identification exercise, 199–200
  My SMART Goals Worksheet exercise, 196–198
SP/SR training. See Self-practice and self-reflection training
Stimulus
  defined, 24
  transfer of stimulus functions, 25–26
  transformation of stimulus functions, 18, 25, 26, 82
Suffering
  the dance between values and suffering, 180–181
  experiential avoidance and, 162–163
Supervisors, working on ACT SP/SR with, 35

Taking the Perspective of My Most Difficult Client (exercise), 141
Thoughts
  inner hooks and the ACT matrix, 99, 102
  separating thoughts from the thinker, 152–153
Time management and planning, 36–37
Time Travel (exercise), 138–140
Tonglen visualization, 227
Tracking behaviors, 29–30
Tracking Intentional Practice: Contacting the Present Moment (exercise), 124
Tracking Opportunities to Practice Willingness and Acceptance (exercise), 170–172
Transcendent self, 85
Transfer of stimulus functions, 25–26
Transformation of stimulus functions, 18, 25, 26, 82

Valued intentions, the challenge problem and, 72

List of Audio Tracks

Track	Title	Run time
1	**Centering** [Chapter 3]	6:11
2	**Self-Practice with Acceptance** [Module 3]	8:19
3	**Self-Practice Contacting the Present Moment** [Module 3]	6:31
4	**Self-Practice with Self-as-Context** [Module 3]	10:27
5	**Self-Practice with Values Authorship** [Module 3]	10:59
6	**Self-Practice with Committed Action** [Module 3]	7:55
7	**Contacting Present-Moment Experience in ACT SP/SR** [Module 5]	14:04
8	**The Ocean of Being** [Module 6]	22:00
9	**Time Travel** [Module 7]	11:28
10	**Externalizing the Thought** [Module 8]	8:06
11	**Dropping the Rope: Letting Go of the Tug-of-War with Our Private Events** [Module 9]	14:20
12	**What Do I Want My Life to Stand For?** [Module 10]	14:28
13	**Exposure** [Module 12]	21:32
14	**Practicing MCA** [Module 13]	15:00
15	**Compassion Circulation** [Module 14]	9:36

The tracks are available to download or stream from The Guilford Press website at *www.guilford.com/tirch2-materials*.

TERMS OF USE